Harvey Bertcher
Linda Farris Kurtz
Alice Lamont
Editors

Rebuilding Communities
Challenges for Group Work

REVIEWS,
COMMENTARIES,
EVALUATIONS . . .

"Traveling globally, *Rebuilding Communities* begins by inviting us to experience the elegant simplicity of a Ghanaian greeting ritual and the respectful silence of a group of Maori New Zealanders. This peaceful sojourn into multicultural group tradition is wisely transformed into the volume's call for a return to social group work's dual focus: individual growth and social goals. A timely and compelling book, *Rebuilding Communities*

provides thoughtful principles for community building and empowerment practice, offers a look at critical areas of group work expertise and 'intelligences,' and describes innovative approaches for addressing some of the most urgent needs of our time. I recommend this fine book to anyone who is ready to meet the challenge of deepening his or her commitment to working with the diverse people and contexts that touch our lives."

Andrew Malekoff, MSW
Director of Program Development,
North Shore Child and Family
Guidance Center,
Roslyn Heights, NY;
Editor, *Social Work with Groups*

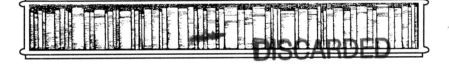

DISCARDED

WIDENER UNIVERSITY

"This book is a collection of papers presented at the Eighteenth Symposium of the Association for the Advancement of Social Work with Groups. The particular papers selected for inclusion in this volume highlight the important role that groups continue to play in confronting contemporary challenges faced by diverse communities everywhere. For example, a keynote presentation on community building reminds the reader that core group work principles are as relevant today as they were a half century ago. However, it is also argued that present-day social problems require us to rethink and reconceptualize our group work practice. Thus, all of the papers reflect the power of groups to build on the strengths of communities, to use community connections and networks to empower individuals, and to improve the quality of life in communities large and small.

Overall, this book is a satisfying read. Each of the authors, in her or his own way, celebrates group work and its ability to unite and empower people from diverse backgrounds and to promote mutual understanding and social and economic justice."

Carolyn Knight, PhD
Associate Professor,
Department of Social Work,
University of Maryland,
Baltimore

"In all, this collection is a fair and effective sampling of the work presented at the Eighteenth Annual Symposium of the Association for the Advancement of Social Work with Groups. It combines the continuing contributions of a group of veteran group workers, both academics and direct practitioners, and an interesting selection of articles by people who are new to this format. The papers consistently are of interest and they are scholarly, well-written, and relevant to today's world and practice. Group work is alive and well, and essential in our current environment. This volume is a fine demonstration of that fact and of the creative work that group workers are doing to help alleviate society's problems and issues."

Robert Salmon, DSW
Professor,
Hunter College School
of Social Work,
New York, NY

"**F**inally, we have an inventive group work book that approaches the topic through a global perspective. Bertcher, Kurtz, and Lamont show how the values and practices of group work have universal applicability.

This book is a testament to the AASWG's achievement in delineating and cementing the bond among group workers worldwide. In this volume, every single chapter has global relevance somewhere else: Berger's groups with immigrant adolescents in the United States, Hanson's research on using groups for AIDS prevention with the mentally ill, and Ramey's presentation of group work's values and broad range of interventions all have utility on virtually every continent.

These papers represent an underlying human rights perspective fostered by the U.N. Declaration of Human Rights, and enacted by humanistic practitioners building groups for mutual support and change within the fabric of caring communities."

Urania Glassman, MSW
Director of Field Instruction,
Wurzweiler School of Social Work,
Yeshiva University

"**R**ebuilding Communities is a landmark in the literature of social work with groups in that almost all of the essays move practice beyond the group into the community. In different ways, they link group work to community organization at either local or global levels, with challenging contributions from social workers in Canada, England, Israel, and South Africa. Presented are multicultural perspectives on the empowerment of people in both geographic communities and those based on bringing together persons with common interests or problems. Practice is now multifaceted, with groups as an integral component of programs that provide essential services and also improve communities. The book provides a rich source of knowledge about contemporary approaches to community-based practice."

Helen Northern, PhD
Distinguished Professor Emerita,
University of Southern California

The Haworth Press, Inc.

Rebuilding Communities
Challenges for Group Work

THE HAWORTH PRESS
Additional Titles of Related Interest

Rebuilding Communities
Challenges for Group Work

Harvey Bertcher
Linda Farris Kurtz
Alice Lamont
Editors

The Haworth Press
New York • London • Oxford

The Haworth Press, Inc., 10 Alice Street, Binghamton, NY 13904-1580

Cover design by Jennifer M. Gaska.

The Library of Congress has cataloged the hardcover edition of this book as:

Rebuilding communities : challenges for group work / Harvey Bertcher, Linda Farris Kurtz, Alice Lamont.
    p.   cm.
    Includes bibliographical references and index.
    ISBN 0-7890-0722-3 (alk. paper).
    1. Social group work. I. Bertcher, Harvey J. II. Kurtz, Linda Farris. III. Lamont, Alice.
HV45.R43 1999
361.4—dc21   99-30672
                                                                  CIP

ISBN 0-7890-0942-0 (pbk.)

CONTENTS

ABOUT THE EDITORS

Harvey Bertcher, MSW, DSW, is Professor Emeritus of social work, School of Social Work, University of Michigan. As a practitioner, he did group work with emotionally disturbed (and disturbing) children, adolescent street gangs, ex-psychiatric hospital patients, and Jewish youth. During his thirty years at Michigan, he taught courses in group work, interpersonal practice, small group theory and role theory, staff development, and social research. His published texts include *Staff Development in Human Service Organizations, Creating Groups* (with Professor Frank Maple), and *Group Participation Techniques for Leaders and Members.* In recent years, he has been particularly interested in group work by telephone. Since the founding of the Association for the Advancement of Social Work with Groups (AASWG), he has taken a leading role in creating songs about group work, accompanying himself on the guitar.

Linda Farris Kurtz, MSW, DPA, is Professor, Department of Social Work, Eastern Michigan University. Her practice experience includes work in a hospital psychiatric clinic, work in an inpatient training and research institute, and responsibility for coordinating a community mental health program. She began her teaching career in 1978, and has taught at the universities of Georgia, Chicago, Indiana, and now Eastern, providing courses in human behavior and the social environment, mental health and substance abuse policy and practice, and social service administration. She is the author of *Self-Help and Support Groups: A Handbook for Practitioners,* and is currently interested in how self-help group participation can lead to political and community action.

Alice Lamont, MSSS, PhD, is Associate Professor Emeritus, having recently retired from the School of Social Work at Wayne State University. Her practice experience includes work at settlement houses and community centers. She also served as coordinator of social services for the Catholic Youth Organization in Detroit. She has taught full time at Wayne State University since 1971, specializing in social work methods and research. Dr. Lamont has written several papers with Ted Goldberg published in the *Journal of Social Work Education* and *Research and Social Group Work,* and in *Roots and New Frontiers in Social Group Work* edited by M. Liederman, M. Birnbaum, and B. Dazzo. Currently, she is coordinator of the MSW program at the School of Social Work. Her recent interests are focused on studying how people learn, with attention to the concept of multiple intelligences.

CONTRIBUTORS

Barbara E. Berger, MSW, is Assistant Professor, Field Liaison, and Supervisor, Department of Social Work, College of St. Catherine, University of St. Thomas, St. Paul, Minnesota.

Roni Berger, PhD, CSW, is Assistant Professor, School of Social Work, Adelphi University, and Group Services in Adolescent Project of JBFCS, Brooklyn, New York.

Karen Culberg, MA, LCSW, was Program Director, Illinois Caucus for Adolescent Health, Chicago, Illinois.[1]

Kendra J. Garrett, DSW, is Associate Professor, Department of Social Work, College of St. Catherine, University of St. Thomas, St. Paul, Minnesota.

Lorraine Gutierrez, PhD, is Associate Professor, School of Social Work, University of Michigan, Ann Arbor, Michigan.

Meredith Hanson, DSW, is Associate Professor, Graduate School of Social Service, Fordham University, New York, New York.

Sue Henry, PhD, is Professor, Graduate School of Social Work, University of Denver, Denver, Colorado.

Lourencia Hofmeyr, PhD, was Senior Lecturer, Department of Social Work, University of Pretoria, Republic of South Africa.[2]

Lea Kacen, PhD, is Department Chair, the Spitzer Department of Social Work, Ben-Gurion University of the Negev, Beersheva, Israel.

Edith A. Lewis, PhD, is Associate Professor of Social Work and Women's Studies, School of Social Work, University of Michigan, Ann Arbor, Michigan.

---

1. Semiretired.
2. Deceased, 1996.

Olga Medina is Director of Latino Affairs, Illinois Caucus for Adolescent Health, Chicago, Illinois.

Audrey Mullender, MA, COSW, is Professor of Social Work, Department of Social Policy and Social Work, University of Warwick, Coventry, England.

Satish K. Nair is a PhD candidate and adjunct faculty member at the Graduate School of Social Work, University of Denver, Denver, Colorado.

Manuel Nakanishi, PhD, is Associate Professor, School of Social Work, Barry University, Miami Shores, Florida.

Arthur J. Naparstek, PhD, is Professor, Mandel School of Applied Social Sciences, Case Western Reserve University, Cleveland, Ohio.

Barbara Neilson, MSW, CSW, is Senior Social Worker, The Hospital for Sick Children, Department of Social Work, Toronto, Ontario, Canada.

Phyllis Pastore, MSW, is Recruitment Training Specialist, Long-Term Care, Jewish and Family Children's Services, West Palm Beach, Florida.

Jennifer Poole, MSW, is Coordinator and Community Worker, Ontario Self-Help Network of Greater Toronto, Toronto, Ontario, Canada.

John H. Ramey, MA, ACSW, LISN, is Associate Professor Emeritus, School of Social Work, University of Akron, Akron, Ohio.

Rebecca Warner, MSN, is Community Health Education Coordinator, Illinois Caucus for Adolescent Health, Chicago, Illinois.

Preface

More than a year ago, I welcomed participants to our eighteenth Symposium on behalf of the Association's Board of Directors. To have the Symposium held at the University of Michigan, the home of many of the profession's group work giants, made it very special for many of us.

I thanked Robert, Alice, and Harvey for lending the Symposium their leadership, tireless effort, and competence. We collectively applauded their amazing accomplishment that was evident in the outstanding program.

A special welcome was extended to international participants and those who were attending their first Symposium.

Finally, I had the privilege of honoring two of our founding members who for more than eighteen years have blessed our Association with their professional vision and competence. In honoring them that evening, we brought honor to ourselves. I stated:

> Professor Katherine Papell, affectionately known to us as Katie. You and Beulah helped with the creation of this association. You and Beulah gave us our very own journal which we look upon with great pride. And while others would rest on their past accomplishments and praises, Katie, you put your energy into the development of the Long Island chapter and serve as its current chair. With great pleasure, I acknowledge your special contributions and what you have meant to us for all these years.
>
> Since the Association began, Professor Ruby Pernell has lent us her competence, style, elegance, and grace. For many of us, Ruby Pernell is as close as we will ever get to royalty. Like Katie, you do not rest on your laurels. You actively participate in the Ohio chapter and provide major leadership to a teen leadership project. On the board, you are our wise sage.

For all you have done for us and for all that you represent, I am very pleased to acknowledge your contributions.

I ended my opening welcome and introductory comments by requesting that I receive an instantaneous and spontaneous outburst of applause.

Now, more than one year later, I am pleased to introduce you to the Symposium Proceedings. It reflects the intellectual vibrancy of the presentations and brings back wonderful memories. I thank the editors for providing us and the profession with this exciting gift.

Alex Gitterman, President
Association for the Advancement
of Social Work with Groups

Acknowledgments

The following people helped to plan and manage the Eighteenth Annual Symposium of the Association for the Advancement of Social Work with Groups: Charlene Anderson, Harvey Bertcher, Debbie Fishman Bierstock, Sallie Churchill, Mary Alice Collins, Bruce Friedman, Charles Garvin, Ted Goldberg, Jane Hassinger, Walter Hill, Alice Lamont, Linda Kurtz, Barbara MacGregor, Tom Morson, Marvin Parnes, John Ramey, Ken Reid, Tom Ruhala, Dan Saunders, Dorothy Seebaldt, Harrison Smith, Dale Swaisgood, Rich Tolman, Robert Williams, and Steve Yanca.

Staff at the University of Michigan, School of Social Work who were particularly helpful included Kitty Foyle and Robin Little.

Staff at the Crowne Plaza who were particularly helpful included Kimberly Hawkins and Karen Ehrheart.

A special note of appreciation must be given to John Ramey. He came all the way from Akron, Ohio, to Ann Arbor to attend every single meeting of the Planning Committee. His input was invaluable.

Introduction

Harvey Bertcher
Linda Farris Kurtz
Alice Lamont

The Eighteenth Annual Symposium of the Association for the Advancement of Social Work with Groups (AASWG) met in Ann Arbor, Michigan, October 24-27, 1996. Ann Arbor is the site of the University of Michigan; two other schools of social work in the immediate area, Eastern Michigan University (in Ypsilanti) and Wayne State University (in Detroit), joined with the University of Michigan's School of Social Work to cosponsor this event.

The Symposium theme, "Rebuilding Communities: Challenges for Group Work," was selected by the Association's Board of Directors. This theme seemed especially appropriate at a time marked by contrasts between regressive responses to social problems, and vibrant examples of community commitment, achieving joint voices linked to community services.

Many of the papers focused on groups in community services or groups serving special client communities. All of the plenary papers included in this volume were concerned with this issue. Arthur Naparstek's paper was a tour de force, linking the history of group work and community organization with current needs. Audrey Mullender spoke convincingly of uniting people through group work on both the local and the global levels. Lorraine Gutierrez and Edith Lewis focused in depth on the interaction of group process with the goal of increasing power through multicultural community work.

The criteria for selecting contributions for this volume included relevance to the Symposium theme, diversity of content, attention to international themes, and a search for authors who had not made presentations at previous Symposia. There were, of course, many veteran contributors and participants whose work continues to enrich group work, but there was also a healthy representation of new contributors, students, and international participants. All of this bodes well for the future of AASWG as an organization.

In the fourteen chapters that follow, the reader will find a rich source of current thinking about group work practice in relation to women, violence, health problems, child welfare, and other areas, as well as group work theory, and the rebuilding of communities through group work processes. As with all of the other symposia from AASWG's rich past, Symposium Eighteen once again made clear that group work is alive and well, and making its contribution to the ongoing effort to solve today's social problems.

SECTION I:
KEYNOTE SPEAKERS

Chapter 1

Strengthening Communities Through Groups: A Multicultural Perspective

Lorraine Gutierrez
Edith A. Lewis

INTRODUCTION

Good afternoon! We welcome you to this luncheon and plenary session. This will be a working session, so we invite you to join with all of us in the collective work. We have been writing about and gathering examples of empowering theory, practice, and research for several years now. We believe that the work of scholars such as Paulo Friere (1970/1994, 1973) has much to teach us in the Western world about practice which increases power, increases access to resources, and informs current structures and processes so that they are improved. These goals of increasing power, increasing access to resources, and improving current structures and processes are key to our understanding of multicultural community work. We believe that this is best done through group processes, so we are very pleased to be working with you as practitioner/scholars of group work.

In our opinion, some of the strongest examples of empowering practice are gleaned from countries other than the United States, and we have attempted to use them to help inform our collaborative work. We will share some of these examples with you today, and have chosen to highlight communities of color in the United States and West Africa.

Goals for This Plenary Session

1. To think collectively about identifying and strengthening our respective communities
2. To understand the role of groups in strengthening communities
3. To develop strategies for strengthening communities through the use of groups

We hope to accomplish these goals through the use of participatory methods (since we are surrounded by wonderful, committed group workers), and to tie these methods to lessons we have learned in our respective practices. We hope that you will be able to utilize some of the methods we have chosen to guide your work together through the remainder of this conference, and in your daily lives as you return to your geographical and psychological communities of choice.

Introductory Exercise

This exercise is designed to help us collectively think about defining the terms "community," "empowerment," and "multiculturalism." On your table, you will find several $3'' \times 5''$ note cards. Please take a card and answer the following questions:

1. How would you define your communities?
2. Which definitions are shared/different at your table?
3. Are those communities multicultural? Why or why not?
4. Would you consider these communities to be empowering? Why or why not?

[Note: After individuals listed their communities, each table then discussed commonalties and differences among their community memberships. Some of these data were collected from all partici- pants in a report-out period at the end of the exercise. Participants found that their perceptions of communities differed greatly. For example, some were concerned about geographic communities, others about communities based on social group memberships (e.g., gay/lesbian/bisexual; age), while others focused on role/status.]

OUR PERSPECTIVE ON COMMUNITY
EMPOWERMENT AND MULTICULTURALISM

Multicultural community empowerment is a term that is commonly used, rarely defined, and often under dispute. It refers to processes that work toward the empowerment of historically disenfranchised groups while creating mechanisms for greater intergroup interaction and change. It is at once pluralistic—and perhaps separatist—and consensus building. It attempts to address the central challenge of living in a diverse society: how do we respect diversity and reduce inequality while working toward a common will? It is built upon a culturally sensitive or culturally competent approach by focusing on efforts to achieve social justice. For example, the goal of multicultural community empowerment is to eliminate the social and economic conditions that encourage young men and women of color to engage in violence and self-destruction.

Multicultural practice methods are grounded in our understanding of culturally sensitive and empowerment-based practice. These are dependent on a set of methods, and also on an orientation to individuals, families, or communities. Central to this perspective include the following three elements:

1. An appreciation and recognition of the strengths existing in communities
2. An understanding of power and how to confront social inequality
3. An understanding of standpoint—how our social location affects what we see in a situation. Where we stand affects what we see. To perform work in a community, we need to understand our own standpoint (and where it comes from) and recognize the standpoint of those around us.

Perspective is particularly important because research on practice has indicated that it is the attitude of the social worker that can have the most impact on outcomes for practice (Gutierrez and Lewis, in press; Reed et al., 1996; Lum, 1996; Figueira-McDonough, Netting, and Nicholas-Casebolt, 1998). To build from strengths, we must recognize and appreciate the strengths in ourselves and those around us. Similarly, if we are to fully appreciate the significance of culture, we need to recognize how our own perspectives have been affected by the world in which we live.

Beyond this perspective, multicultural practice within groups and communities requires the ability to carry out the methods of empowering practice that have been found to be effective for increasing the power of individuals, families, and communities (Gutierrez and Lewis, in press). Research suggests that empowering practice is built upon methods that are educational, participatory, and capacity building (Minkler, 1997; Adams, Bell, and Griffin, 1997).

Educational methods are focused on working with participants to develop the ability to understand and act upon the social environment. The focus of these methods is on understanding one's situation and community and to develop skills to increase one's own interpersonal or political power. Consciousness-raising methods can be used to help groups and communities understand the nature of their problems. This understanding can also clarify possible responses or solutions to difficult situations.

Education also involves the development of specific skills to address power deficits and develop greater resources. These skills can include formal training on such information as immigrant rights, or on skills such as conflict management. It can also include assertiveness training, time management, skills for running a meeting, or an analysis of the political process.

The *participatory methods* utilized in multicultural empowerment efforts require working collaboratively within groups and communities. They involve recognizing and sharing one's own power in order to develop the power of others. When doing this work we must perceive ourselves as enablers, organizers, consultants, or compatriots with communities and groups in an effort to avoid replicating the powerlessness experience with other helpers or professionals. We must presume that we do not hold the "answers" to problems, but that in the context of collaboration, community members will develop the insights, skills, and capacity to resolve their own situations. The organizer is at the service of the community, not the other way around.

In building capacity, we start with strengths and work from there. Our focus is on abilities and strengths, not on problems and deficiencies. We see what is working and how that can be used to gain more power. A capacity-building perspective recognizes that individuals and communities have been operating in oppressive circumstances that have inhibited their ability to act effectively. Our role is to develop strategies to address the oppressive circumstance.

One example of operationalizing a capacity-building model comes from an experience in which a group of undergraduate students visited a Head Start center in Detroit. These undergraduates were struck by the physical deterioration and poverty of the surrounding neighborhood and the positive energy within the center. The center was a section of a church basement, partitioned off by temporary walls. The staff, all of whom came from the neighborhood, showed considerable caring when interacting with the children.

In a question-and-answer period after the tour, one student asked: "How would you describe this neighborhood?" The center director replied: "This is a very strong neighborhood. There are some real resources here—churches, good neighborhood schools, a WIC center down the block, close families. Parents here are involved with the center—over 60 percent of our employees are volunteers. Some blocks have strong associations that work together on crime prevention, gardening, clean ups, and so on."

The students were impressed by the strengths-based approach of the center director. Although the poverty of this neighborhood was apparent, her view was of a resilient and vibrant community.

You've experienced the elements of multicultural community empowerment with the first exercise we did this afternoon. Rather than define the types of communities you potentially belonged to, we elicited that information from you, the experts on your communities. We utilized participatory and educational methods commonly used in groups to engage you in capacity building with one another. Now we'd like to give you some additional examples of multicultural empowerment within groups that we've experienced recently. We hope that these will further illustrate the principles of consciousness raising, capacity building, and connection or collaboration.

EXAMPLES OF MULTICULTURAL
EMPOWERMENT IN GROUPS

Examples from Ghana—Edith Lewis's Stories

Specific Attention to Difference in the Composition
of Subcommittees, Committees, Neighborhoods

Group theory and practice in the United States suggests that we must pay attention to issues of group composition in order to maximize group outcomes (Gutierrez et al., 1998; Lewis and Ford, 1990; Chau, 1992; Brower et al., 1987). The multicultural literature further suggests to us that recognizing difference in groups helps us to avoid the pitfalls of erroneously assuming homogeneity in the midst of potentially critical heterogeneity. The empowerment literature recommends that we not only recognize but embrace the differences among group members so that all are involved in expanding their processes of critical consciousness through connection with others.

During Fulbright studies in Ghana, West Africa, in 1995, I had the opportunity to witness in many arenas the operationalization of a multicultural, empowering approach to group composition. For example, at meetings in the Viva Ghana Consortium of child welfare agencies in the Greater Accra region, much of the consortium's work was distributed among subcommittees. As each subcommittee's task was outlined, and members volunteered to participate, an interesting phenomenon occurred. Before moving on to the next agenda item, someone within the group would specifically draw the group's attention to the composition of the subcommittee. We would become engaged in an exercise to ensure that we had considered the ratio of men to women in the group, representation from secular and religious bodies with different ideological perspectives, official nongovernmental organizations versus groups without that governmental recognition, and groups with extensive resources versus those truly operating on shoestring budgets. Even more interesting, those individuals raising the questions in the majority of cases were not those fewer women with the group, nor those from smaller religious/secular groups, nor those with limited governmental status or resources. Instead, the questions about representation were made by those who would have been considered to have power, and their interest in balance was genuine. They had learned, it appears, that conscious attention to difference enhances rather than detracts, can help groups understand the complexities and "unintended consequences" of a set of actions, and provides opportunities for increased knowledge development for all members.

What would happen if we in the United States could learn from this lesson about group composition? What would happen if group workers and group and community members consciously attended to group composition on an ongoing basis through the life of the group? What would happen if, before any decision was finalized, the group engaged in a discussion of that decision's "unintended consequences" for all represented with the community? Wouldn't "welfare reform" look a lot different than it does now if group composition and difference had been attended to? Wouldn't the tenure and promotion status of women in the academy look a lot different if group composition and difference had been attended to? Wouldn't we have moved beyond the "affirmative action" stage of ethnic group relationships, had group composition and difference been attended to?

Greeting Rituals As a Form of Building Community
with Divergent Groups

When one begins a conversation for the first time in a day with a Ghanaian, one must first greet the individual. Usually, this is done on the street with a simple "Good morning," "Good afternoon," or "Good evening." Not to greet another individual is considered the height of incivility, and many expatriates will explain this by telling you that Ghana was a British colony and that they have adopted the British civility code.

I beg to differ on this point, because the greeting ritual is far more complex than this, particularly when visiting a Ghanaian home or having someone visit your home. The first order of business is the greeting ritual, which employs pouring water, shaking the hands of all visitors, welcoming them, and asking them about their purpose for visiting. To breech any part of this ritual can be considered rude. I (Edith) did not understand how rude the behavior was considered until the father of one of my friends came in from a distant village and was brought to meet me during my first month in the country.

While I poured the water and presented it to him, I did not move to shake his hand and the hands of those accompanying him immediately. He told his son (who was translating for us) that he wished to be "greeted in the traditional way." Once this was done, he relaxed and began to offer me a wealth of information that I would not have been privy to had I not been able to engage in this activity.

What does this have to do with group work? The ritual of greeting extends to social welfare and human rights organizations throughout Ghana. For example, the Consortium of Women Organizations in the capital city of Accra, has representatives from forty-five different groups. Some are Muslim, some Christian. Some represent attorneys, bankers, nurses, community organizers, and nongovernmental organizations. Many of these women do not encounter one another at any time other than the group meetings. Sometimes attendance at these meetings tops 100 women. Nonetheless, the greeting ritual of shaking hands with other women attending the meeting occurs, no matter how long it takes!!! It is important, before attending to the business at hand, that all participants are welcomed and that their presence is recognized.

This lesson was one of my favorites because it helped me understand how some rituals survived the Middle Passage (i.e., the Atlantic slave trade), and continue to be exhibited in Africans across the diaspora. Some of these same greeting rituals are seen in churches on Sunday mornings, at family reunions, at the Association of Black Social Workers conferences across the country, and during Mardi Gras in New Orleans. Now I ask you to participate in the ritual. Turn to those at the table around you and shake their hands, and truly welcome them! Turn to those you can reach at the table across from you and do the same. Make the connection with one another!

Taking the Time to Translate into Multiple Languages
at Formal Programs

Ghanaians recognize that although their official language is English, many ethnic groups are represented, and several languages are spoken throughout the country. Therefore Ghanaian citizens, as most individuals in the world outside of the United States, are at least bilingual, and often multilingual. This realization became apparent as I watched the three-year-old son of the woman who worked at my house effortlessly move among three languages, depending upon with whom he was speaking. At three, this small child, not financially privileged nor yet in school, was able to communicate with many different children and adults, and learn from all of them. He was also, for example, the bridge between the two children in our compound who had been born in Massachusetts, and were able to speak only English, and whose peer-aged cousins would tease them unmercifully by speaking in Ga or Twi. Certainly, my determination to be able to perform the basic greetings in both Twi and Ga, and to further polish my Spanish and German grew after encountering this young man!

The nation we live in continues to be one in which bilingualism is not required, must less celebrated. What would happen if we were happy that our taxi driver spoke multiple languages instead of muttering under our breaths that he should "learn good English!!!" Would recognizing standard dialects such as occur among some African Americans living in close proximity to one another or some American Indian tribes whose original tongues have been greatly modified through the years provide us with an expanded awareness of how the world is constructed for different communities? Would our multilingual children be able to move beyond the quotas now used to ensure ethnic representation, to the building of new experiences gleaned from a new common language?

Lest we think that these examples would only be possible in a group- and community-oriented country such as Ghana, we have other examples found here in the United States.

Examples from the United States—Lorraine Gutierrez's Stories

The People of Color Against AIDS Network (POCAAN)

POCAAN is an intercommunity interorganizational coalition of color in Seattle, Washington. POCAAN was originally organized in opposition to existing AIDS/HIV prevention and treatment groups that were not focused on this population. This organization is structured around group development by providing grants to specific ethnic communities to carry out their own programs. The focus is on community development through such organizations as the

Brother to Brother Network for Gay Men of Color, Sister to Sister for women of color, and focusing work in churches and other faith-based groups.

POCAAN's overarching theme is building community through groups. For example, they bring together gay black men to gather information, provide social support, develop campaigns and carry out work. The work involves group support and community organizing. This work can then involve other groups such as the Latino Network which can conduct coordinated peer health education, needle exchange, and so forth. POCAAN becomes the source of support, ideas, and action.

The Association for the Advancement of Social Work with Groups (AASWG)

AASWG is another example. Taking the advice of Mother Jones ("Don't mourn, organize") the founders of this organization responded to the marginalization and underrepresentation of group work at various national NASW and CSWE conferences, by forming our own independent organization and holding our own conferences separate from the official bodies of the profession or academia.

We have grown our own organization through local chapters and meetings at other conferences (which often resembled small groups). I'd like to believe that our background as group workers has made us particularly effective in organizing ourselves and making a difference to our profession. It has resulted in a viable organization and also some research and activism that has had an impact on CSWE, NASW, and social work research, teaching, and practice.

How Do These Examples Add to Our Knowledge of Multicultural Community Empowerment?

Several lessons can be learned from these five examples of multicultural community empowerment. They may be summarized as follows:

1. It is important to recognize and utilize existing networks and rituals (as in the example of POCAAN, and the greeting custom preceding formal and informal gatherings in Ghana).

2. Multicultural community-empowering group workers are multi-lingual and multicultural (as in the example for Ghana.)
3. Community members must define and develop their own structures, as in the example from AASWG. (Think of what would happen if CSWE told us how to hold our meetings or structure our local chapters!)
4. Difference can be recognized and incorporated as a strength rather than a weakness in multicultural community-empowerment work (as illustrated by the case of Ghanaian social welfare consortia.)

COMMITMENT

Our definition of empowering practice requires not just a change in the ways we think about ourselves as members of communities, but also requires one to act on the different information. We have designed a way for you to operationalize empowering practice within your community while participating in this plenary session. In other words, we are going to ask you to follow the Ghanaian example of group work within communities and tax yourselves. We want to ask you to think for a moment about what one activity you can commit yourself to within the next six months as a way of strengthening your community. Remember, all contributions to strengthening communities, no matter how small, may be useful. Write your commitment on one of the sheets of paper provided at each table. Now, please take an envelope from the center of the table and address it to yourself. Now that you have identified your commitment to your community for the next six months, give your envelope to someone else at your table. In six months that person is responsible for mailing it back to you. That person is holding your commitment for the next six months. Although this person does not know the secrets contained in your envelope, he or she has joined with you to further that commitment by sharing the information with you. Please don't forget to send one another the envelopes by April 25, 1997.

CLOSING

What we have attempted to do in this plenary session is to use participatory methods to highlight some of the basic principles of

empowerment practice in groups. We have also attempted to operationalize these principles with case examples from our own experience as well as having you operationalize the principles in some
meaningful way in your own lives. We hope that this presentation
has been helpful, wish you a good day, and a good remainder of the
conference. Thank you for your participation.

REFERENCES

Adams, Maurianne, Bell, Lee Anne, and Griffin, Pat, Eds. (1997). *Teaching for Diversity and Social Justice: A Sourcebook.* New York: Routledge.
Brower, Aaron, M., Garvin, Charles D., Hobson, Josephine, Reed, Beth G., and Reed, Harvey (1987). Exploring the effects of leader gender and race on group behavior. In Lassner, J., Powell, K., and Finnigan, E. (Eds.), *Social Group Work: Competence and Values in Practice.* Binghamton, NY: The Haworth Press, Inc., 129-148.
Chau, K. (1992). Needs assessment for group work with people of color: A conceptual formulation. *Social Work with Groups,* 15(2/3), 53-66.
Figueira-McDonough, Josefina, Netting, F. Ellen, and Nicholas-Casebolt, Ann (Eds.) (1998). *The Role of Gender in Practice Knowledge: Claiming Half the Human Experience.* New York: Garland.
Friere, Paulo (1970/1994). *Pedagogy of the Oppressed (Revised Edition).* New York: Continuum.
Friere, Paulo (1973). *Education for Critical Consciousness.* New York: Seabury.
Gutierrez, Lorraine and Lewis, Edith (in press). *Empowering Social Work Practice with Women of Color.* New York: Columbia.
Gutierrez, Lorraine, Reed, Beth, Ortega, Robert, and Lewis, Edith (1998). Teaching about groups in a gendered world: Toward curricular transformation in group work education. In Figueira-McDonough, J., Nichols-Casebolt, A., and Netting, F. (Eds.), *The Role of Gender in Practice Knowledge.* New York: Garland, 170-204.
Lewis, Edith and Ford, B. (1990). The network utilization project: Incorporating traditional strengths of African-American families into group work practice. *Social Work with Groups,* 13(3), 7-22.
Lum, Doman (1996). *Social Work Practice and People of Color: A Process-Stage Approach,* Third Edition. Pacific Grove, CA: Brooks/Cole.
Minkler, Meredith (Ed.) (1997). *Community Organization and Community Building for Health.* New Brunswick, NJ: Rutgers.
Reed, Beth G., Newman, Peter A., Suarez, Zulema E., and Lewis, Edith A. (1996). Interpersonal practice beyond diversity and towards social justice: The importance of critical consciousness. In Garvin, G. and Seabury, B. (Eds.), *Interpersonal Practice,* Second Edition. Englewood Cliffs, NJ: Prentice-Hall, 44-76.

Chapter 2

Community Building and Social Group Work: A New Practice Paradigm for American Cities

Arthur J. Naparstek

I became a social group worker thirty-five years ago because I felt then, as I do today, that we have become a society that has lost its capacity for compassion. Seemingly overwhelmed by our responsibilities, we are leaning more and more toward the approach that if something can't be fixed, ignore the problem. I am guided by the values and belief systems of the great social movements of my life: the Civil Rights Movement, the Labor Movement, the Settlement House Movement, the Peace Movement, and the Women's Movement.

We have to return to the roots of these social movements and demand that the government lead the way to equal opportunity. We must again demand that the government build a role in support of families and communities, and that the government must provide:

- The moral leadership to bring out the best in this country
- The legal framework to ensure equal opportunity, access, and equity
- The tools for community self-help and initiative

It is our responsibility to make it happen.

We are living in tough times. They are tough times economically and socially and they are tough times for social programs. And, these are very tough times for poor people.

For years, I believed that we would gradually see the poor moving toward a better life. But we see that exactly the opposite has happened. Not only have the poor not found a better life, but the working class have become downwardly mobile; many are the new poor, and their numbers are growing. Demagogues are now appealing to this group.

Many examples of great changes are sweeping America, such as President Clinton signing the welfare reform bill; the new form of nativism best represented by the anti-immigration sentiment in California; the strength of the Christian Coalition; the threatened rollback of abortion rights and gay rights; the movement toward creationism; the implied anti-city and anti-minority feelings; much of which is implicit in the policies of the "so-called" devolution revolution.

We are experiencing a long, painful transition to a post-industrial economy. The economic problems can be contained in a word: poverty. Behind every number, behind all the data, you find people.

Two out of three adults living in poverty are women with children. Many of them are the working poor. They are waitresses. They are clerks. They live from paycheck to paycheck, without services for child care, prenatal care, nutrition. Others come from the ranks of those who were beginning to get ahead in the days of affirmative action. Those days are gone and so are the jobs.

I've seen shelters for women in cities throughout Ohio. In the past, these were intended as overnight shelters for battered women. But something has happened. Young women have been turning up with their preschool children, women who once had jobs and homes. These shelters are inundated with the new poor.

We need to understand why our national solutions have never worked as well as they should. There are no simple solutions. From income maintenance to community development block grants, programs look at poverty as if it were a single, seamless problem, unrelated to other forces and amenable to monolithic solutions parachuted in from somewhere above. In the inability to see that it is impossible to change one element in an open system without altering all the others, we have failed to see that our solutions, while well-intentioned, create negative preconditions and make it impossible for anything to work.

For example, we have learned that income maintenance can be a disincentive to work. Public housing can and often has created ghettos, and public education has not dealt with the needs of inner-city children. In cities such as Cleveland, families and neighborhoods have changed as more children have only one parent in their homes, and because women and/or both parents are working, there are fewer and fewer people in the neighborhood. Yet, the urban systems serving these neighborhoods have yet to change. The problems of Cleveland and cities like it are at a critical point.

Systems that serve the poor and minorities need to be reexamined. For example, public welfare, public housing, and public education were organized to meet problems and needs that are different from those found in today's urban minority community. Each system serves as a vehicle of alienation rather than a stimulus for mobility or a supporter of individual and family life. The public schools in Cleveland were redefined at the turn of the century to meet the needs of the children of eastern and southern European immigrants in a newly industrialized city; the Department of Human Services was an outgrowth of the Great Depression and designed to meet the needs of people who were thought to be temporarily caught in the economic dislocation of the times; and public housing, which originated in Cleveland in 1935—Cedar Estates—and was meant to be temporary housing, was targeted for the worker dislocated by the Depression or the white widow with two children.

The 1994 congressional campaign, which gave America the contract and the 1996 presidential campaign, is forcing us to begin this reexamination. The process of reexamination suggests we return to the roots of our profession, particularly the values that served as the basis for social group work. I was particularly moved by a recent re-reading of a paper by Grace Coyle delivered in 1935 to the National Conference on Social Welfare (Coyle, 1947). The relevance of the paper to contemporary time can be found in her opening statement. She said:

> In a period like the present, every human activity must test itself by its contribution to the vital changes that are making our society. Group work is a part of the educational process by which society aims to produce certain effects in individuals

and to preserve and transform its cultural heritage. . . . Group work has several purposes and the interpretation of its functions will vary from agency to agency and from worker to worker. Certain of its purposes aim at the growth and adjustment of the individual. (Coyle, 1947, p. 142)

But, like all education, it also cannot avoid social responsibility for the making of citizens, that is, for the production in individuals of those attitudes and accomplishments that will contribute to the kind of society we desire. I believe her work serves as a basis for this reexamination.

Today, we should be arguing for a paradigm shift. A paradigm is a framework of thought—a scheme for understanding and explaining certain aspects of reality. A paradigm shift is a distinctly new way of thinking about old problems. A new paradigm involves a principle that was present all along but unknown to us.

In making the shift, we need to build on the work of Coyle, but current demands necessitate the need to conceptualize the process somewhat differently. We have to become what the economist and educator Robert Theobald calls weavers.

A weaver is someone who designs open networks, who sees patterns and connections, making the network more effective. The network is the most powerful social form of our time, a new king of open system, a community so coherent in its value that it can withstand and even welcome the constant flow of events. The network is a process, a moving vehicle for community building (Ferguson, 1990). The aspect of the paradigm shift that I would like to talk about is networking in the context of building strong communities.

COMMUNITY BUILDING: WHAT IS IT?

What do community builders do? Joan Walsh in an unpublished report to the Rockefeller Foundation notes that the approaches are diverse and locally tailored: in Denver, black churches have dramatically expanded their work with low-income families, thanks to an innovative partnership with local and national funders. In the South Bronx, five community development corporations have created an employment network to do whatever it takes—from résumé writing to conflict resolution—to connect area residents to the mainstream labor market. In Savannah, Georgia, a high-powered collaborative is testing new ways to deliver services and engage residents in the city's poorest neighborhoods. In Baltimore, paid community advocates tied to a comprehensive health, housing, and economic development initiative are rebuilding a once-devastated neighborhood, block by block. In Atlanta, a corporation partnering with community residents is turning a high school into a much-needed family resource center.

Walsh writes that the roster of community-building boosters is equally diverse. HUD Secretary Henry Cisneros is a believer, weaving community building principles into new federal policy for public housing and economic development, especially the landmark $2 billion Empowerment Zone/Enterprise Community initiative, and the $2.6 billion HOPE VI Initiative that was sponsored by Senator Barbara Mikulski of Maryland. But so is Newt Gingrich, who has pushed community-building strategies to revitalize Washington, DC. Supporters include urban self-help advocate John McKnight, who wants to dismantle most of the social welfare state; the Children's Defense Fund, which advocates reform and expansion of services; and the Committee for Economic Development, an influential corporate think tank whose 1995 report on community building made a bottom line case for business to form partnerships with neighborhoods to rebuild American cities. Conservative columnist George Will visited Baltimore's Community Building in Partnership and came away a partisan, describing it as a model of Jeffersonian democracy (Walsh, 1996).

Community building consists, quite simply, of encouraging activities that enhance the ability of people to work together for a common purpose in groups or organizations. It is only when people feel some measure of control over their fates, feel that they have the ability to set standards that will be enforced, sense that they share common assets—and have a stake in their proper investment, indeed, have the ability to determine community priorities—that community, true community, is born, and with it, the ability to accomplish their individual and shared goals.

In a community building approach, private citizens and public systems come together in joint endeavors that are conceived, planned, and implemented on the small scale we commonly think of as the local community or neighborhood. It is, after all, in neighborhoods where the best opportunity exists for people to claim ownership of the processes that could help them regain some control over their lives.

Certainly the idea of community-based interventions is not new to social work or to work in low-income neighborhoods. Community development has roots in nineteenth-century utopian and communitarian thought, and in the later initiatives of twentieth-century black leaders and community activists. Comprehensive community strategies were also part and parcel of the settlement house movement of the late nineteenth century and more recently these strategies reemerged in the War on Poverty programs of the 1960s and the community development work of the past twenty years (Connell et al., 1995). For social work practice, community has been central for more than one hundred years.

Spergal (1972), Rubin and Rubin (1992), Garvin and Cox (1995) all identify major periods in the development of community organization practice. These authors provide a broad overview of the social, political, and cultural forces that have defined the various periods or eras of community organization practice.

However, events of the past two decades have stimulated the development of new approaches to community intervention. One emerging approach sets forth a long-term strategy for addressing the issues confronting inner-city neighborhoods. It builds on the assumption that poverty is the single biggest cause of the deterioration of a neighborhood's social fabric, and that the best way to improve urban neighborhoods is to reduce poverty through a community-building process.

Two major factors influenced the recent development of community-building as a field of practice. First, the early 1980s saw a host of changes in federal policy. President Reagan put the nation on a fundamentally different course, reducing the federal role in eight areas: income security, health, social services, transportation, housing and community development, employment, training and economic development, and education.

As a result, changes in three broad thematic areas emerged: the shifting of responsibility to state and local governments; a greater reliance on the private sector and the mechanisms of the market; and a narrower targeting of benefits to individuals (Palmer and Sawhill, 1982).

Stimulated by these changes and the resultant budget cuts in human service programs and delivery systems, communities throughout the nation began to debate how best to restructure human service delivery systems. State, local, and national governments, along with foundation executives and policy analysts, recognize the need for new ways of thinking about and responding to poverty. The result has been a movement toward community-based intervention strategies.

Often directed by community residents, these efforts have focused on child welfare reform, family preservation with at-risk families, and housing and economic development. They differ from past strategies in several important respects. First, these initiatives seek to bridge the gap between human services and physical revitalization, including housing and economic development; second, they focus on enhancing neighborhood leadership and mobilizing broad participation in the revitalization effort; and third, they attempt to create links between various programs so that families and individuals are seen in holistic ways.

The second major change factor that influenced community building came from a ground-breaking research study in which Professor William Julius Wilson (Wilson, 1991) documented the internal dynamics of several poor Chicago neighborhoods, suggesting that persistent poverty—the kind of poverty that endures over many years and, with increasing frequency, is passed from one generation to another—is concentrated in geographic areas. He found this kind of poverty in neighborhoods marked by a deteriorating social infrastructure, with fraying or absent networks of churches, schools, banks, businesses, neighborhood centers, and families. The connection between dedicated social support systems and persistent poverty was established; conversely, Wilson also demonstrated the correlation between a strong community and the ability of its residents to get out of poverty (Wilson, 1991). I will come back to this point later in the chapter.

In response to these two factors, human service agencies and foundations began to seek new ways of thinking about and responding to poverty. During the decade of the eighties, the Ford, Annie Casey, and Rockefeller foundations initiated major community-building programs, often in partnership with community foundations, and state and county human service agencies (Eisen, 1992). Foundation initiatives responded to the following trends.

Reverse Fragmentation/Categorization

In the 1970s, integration was developed as a top-down strategy for managing human service programs. Interest in the concept waned during the Reagan years, but has recently reemerged in a somewhat different configuration—for example, now cutting across agency lines and programs dealing with children and families that have failed in their fragmented categorized approach to address the inter-related causes of poverty (Melaville and Blank, 1991).

Human service professionals have recognized that fragmentation and categorical social service programs and supports are limiting program success. Criticisms leveled against human services have included: lack of coordination of services; fragmentation of services; inaccessibility of services; problems of accountability; barriers to care and effective intervention by professionals; and a lack of understanding of community (Naparstek, Biegel, and Spiro, 1982).

Cutting across all of these issues is the fact that internal community-helping systems are not recognized, not utilized, and do not form an integrated service resource. Although knowledge exists about neighborhood-helping networks, they never have been sufficiently utilized to address the issues of fragmentation and lack of accessibility and accountability.

Place-Based/People-Based Intervention Strategies

Community development experts now recognize that, with some notable exceptions, physical revitalization had come to dominate activities on the ground, but that "bricks and mortar interventions" alone do not achieve sustained improvement in low-income neighborhoods. While physical development is an essential element and a logical starting point, for many practitioners, funders, and policymakers, "community development" has come to mean influencing community life along many dimensions—physical, social, economic, individual, institutional, and political. The challenge is to combine a focus on places with people-based strategies. For example, "people" strategies many relate to the plight of children in poverty and the reform of the welfare system; while "place" strategies focus on such issues as housing, economic development, and commercial revitalization.

Linking place- and people-based strategies through comprehensive community building means improving the delivery and quality of human services, strengthening community organization, stimulating economic development, and in every possible way, improving the quality of life while affecting physical improvements. Over the years, numerous public and philanthropic initiatives have addressed such concerns as poverty, welfare, unemployment, inadequate education, substantial housing and crime. But past efforts have tended to consider these problems one at a time. People/place-based strategies address the crucial fact that the coexistence of problems within a neighborhood creates a mutually reinforcing process of decay that limits the effectiveness of narrowly focused initiatives (Svirdoff, 1994).

THE APPROACH:
HOW DOES COMMUNITY BUILDING WORK?

In the light of fresh thinking about urban neighborhoods and the new, hard-won insights into the nature of urban poverty, four general principles have emerged that describe and guide community-building initiatives. It is these four principles, taken together, that make this approach distinctive and maximize its chances for success.

Community-Building Principles

Principle I: Community Building Is Comprehensive and Integrative

Poverty-related problems are interlocking and overlapping. Yet previous attempts to combat poverty have ignored this fact, isolating specific problems, such as housing or job training, for intensive intervention. Research shows, for example, that a relationship exists between the proliferation of female-headed households, the persistence of poverty over two or more generations, the concentration of poor households in the inner city, and quality-of-life issues such as health care and poor outcomes for school-aged children. If one is to deal with the issue of female-headed households, unemployment— particularly male unemployment—must be addressed, because the shortage of "marriageable" males in the inner city is directly related to the shortage of employed males. If existing transportation systems are not getting inner-city residents to where the work is, or if the available jobs require a different level of skills from what is available in the community, efforts directed merely at employment are of little use. Similarly, it does little good to offer a young inner-city mother a job if she lacks proper day care for her children, or adequate health care coverage, or is struggling with other problems in her family that continually deplete her energies and drag her down (Coulton, 1989).

Unfortunately, the social service system as it is currently set up tends to isolate and address various needs as if they were unrelated. Areas of need such as housing or jobs are typically addressed, for example, as if they had nothing to do with health or education.

Housing projects become prisons for the poor and the elderly when issues of crime and security, or city services are not also addressed. But the entire system of human services is set up in such a way as to separate all these issues—children's needs from the needs of their parents, health care from job training, food stamps from completing an education. Each system has evolved its own separate bureaucracy and set of hoops for people to jump through. When systems don't acknowledge these links and fail to act with the bigger picture in mind, failure is inevitable.

A community-building approach to alleviating poverty acknowledges the interconnectedness of problems confronting families, and recommends a course of action in which solutions are tied together.

Principle II: Community Building Takes Advantage
of the New Forms of Collaboration and Partnership
by Strengthening Community-Based Networks

Because government's role is changing, new ways of proceeding through collaborative decision making are being developed. The movement toward devolution of program authority from federal to local levels (state and county) through block grants puts substantial pressure on local health, education, and social service agencies to meet local needs. Through devolution of authority to lower levels of government, the federalism of the 1990s is intended to stimulate innovations in service delivery, streamline bureaucracy, and reduce dependency. The key to making this devolution process work—advocates of the community-building approach believe—is the movement away from the categorical approach toward comprehensive block grants.

In effect, devolution is both a "top-down" and a "bottom-up" process. Experience has shown that either an exclusively top-down or a bottom-up approach to alleviating poverty is inadequate. An exclusively "top-down" strategy lacks significant contributions from practitioners, stakeholders, and the intended beneficiaries. On the other hand, approaches that are solely "bottom-up," though often effective for building support for single issues, are less likely to produce the comprehensive policy changes that are needed to address more complex realities. Decision-making efforts that concentrate on achieving a full consensus are frequently characterized by "least common denominator" thinking. In an attempt to reach a consensus, these efforts often fail to raise the level of discussion.

Successful strategies borrow effective aspects of each approach by combining leadership and potential for large-scale impact with the impending nature of community-driven initiatives. This new form of collaboration is guided by a strategy that strengthens the traditional source of support in communities: families, churches, social clubs, and other voluntary associations.

In many poor communities informal support and networks that help people are not as effective as they could be. Local people must be actively involved in shaping community-building strategies. Different neighborhoods have different needs and meet their needs in different ways. Only by engaging people can the networks become energized.

Alexis de Tocqueville attributed the success of democracy in America to a national propensity for civic engagement. Robert Putnam (1993) points out that recent empirical research in a wide range of contexts has confirmed that the norms and networks of civic engagement can improve education, diminish poverty, inhibit crime, boost economic performance, foster better governments, and even reduce mortality rates. Conversely, deficiencies in a community-based network contribute to a wide range of social, economic, and political ills. Putnam's review of the literature demonstrates the extent to which scholars and practitioners who are concerned about urban poverty and joblessness have similarly focused on the role of community networks and norms. He notes that although the empirical verdict is not yet complete, one careful study by Anne Case and Lawrence Katz (1992) of the prospects of youths in Boston illustrates the phenomenon that has attracted so much attention. Controlling for all relevant individual characteristics (such as race, gender, education, parental education, family structure, religious involvement, and so on), youth whose neighbors attend church are more likely to have jobs, less likely to use drugs, and less likely to be involved in criminal activity. In other words, church-going (the most common form of civic engagement in America) has important "externalities," in the sense that it influences the behavior and life prospects of "bystanders," whether they themselves are so engaged. Similarly, research on the varying economic attainments of different ethnic groups in the United States has demonstrated the importance of social bonds within each group. These results are consistent with research in a wide range of settings that demonstrate the vital importance of social networks for job placement and many other economic outcomes. Putnam also points out that, a seemingly unrelated body of research on the sociology of economic development (Borlias, 1992) has also focused attention on the role of social networks. Some of this work is situated in the developing countries, and some of it elucidates the peculiarly successful "network capitalism," of East Asia. Even in less exotic Western economies, however, researchers have discovered highly efficient, highly flexible "industrial districts," based on networks of collaboration among workers and small entrepreneurs. Far from being paleoindustrial anachronisms, these dense interpersonal and interorganizational networks undergird ultramodern industries, from the high tech of Silicon Valley to the high fashion of Benetton (Putnam, 1993).

In the field of education, researchers have discovered that successful schools are distinguished not so much by the control of their curriculum or the quality of their teachers as by their embeddedness in a broader fabric of supportive families and communities. James S. Coleman and T. B. Hoffer (1987) found that the success of private schools is attributable less to what happens in the classroom or to the endowments of individual students than to the greater engagement of parents and community members in school activities. James Comer (1980), an educational psychologist seeking to revitalize American public schools in disadvantaged communities, has shown the power of strategies that involve parents and community members in the educational process.

Social epidemiologists have shown that social ties have consequences even for physical morbidity and mortality. An as-yet unpublished study of the comparative effectiveness of anti-AIDS interventions among at-risk populations (prostitutes, IV drug users, teenage runaways, and so on) in various American communities, for example, seems to show that a given program will be substantially more effective when the target population, no matter how disconnected from the larger society, is characterized by greater internal connectedness. Other research on the general population has found that people with comparatively few social and community ties face substantially greater risks of physical and mental illness and mortality, controlling for socioeconomic status and for physiological risk factors. One study, for example, found that controlling for factors of sex, age, race, socioeconomic status, physical health, and personal hygiene, social connectedness lowered mortality risk by more than half. Joining, in short, is good for your health (Putnam, 1993).

Principle III: Community Building
Builds on Neighborhood Assets

Past efforts have failed to link services and development initiatives to the asset base of a community. Human service practitioners have traditionally focused on a deficit or need-based approach to those being served. John McKnight offers a different strategy for empowering low-income communities, starting with the idea that poor neighborhoods also have assets. He likens it to viewing the glass as half full instead of half empty. He argues that mental health, human services, and community and economic development initiatives are more likely to succeed if based on the strengths, resources, and diversities existing in local communities (Kretzmann and McKnight, 1993).

Indeed, empirical evidence now supports the efficacy of community-based assets. Robert Putnam's comparative study of communities in northern and southern Italy has revealed that such organizations as guilds, religious fraternities, cooperatives, mutual aid societies, and neighborhood associations are preconditions for economic development (Putnam, 1993).

Two kinds of existing community associations are suited to the job of building a neighborhood's assets and capacities. One is the multi-issue community organization, built along coalition lines. Community organizers understand the importance of associational life to the well-being of neighborhoods. Another is the Community Development Corporation. The Community Development Corporation's distinguishing characteristics are the comprehensive nature of its purpose and its flexibility. Many CDCs work with a range of neighborhood-based assets such as small business, commercial ventures, and finance and housing, often relying on a social-planning approach.

Principle IV: Community Building Targets Neighborhoods
to Enhance Resident Participation

When specific neighborhoods are targeted for interventions, residents become more involved in shaping strategies. The temptation is often to attack the problem of poverty by going citywide or metropolitan, but we now know that such macro approaches are doomed. It is at the neighborhood level that people feel the consequences of policy and planning decisions. Residents have knowledge about their neighborhoods and that is an essential ingredient to a responsive planning effort. Their values, their insights, and their needs, as they perceive them, must be incorporated into any meaningful process.

A small-scale focus also minimizes the possibilities of unintended consequences of the sort that can result from defining a program for broad application in a wide variety of circumstances.

Community building involves many intangible forces, such as informal networks of support and leadership, that are critical to any long-term efforts. Such relationships need to be nurtured and encouraged as part of the process. Any effort directed at changing systems and social structures must focus on a distinct geographic area whose residents are linked by, and who identify with, a cluster of local institutions such as schools, churches, or community centers. Key to all is that in place of structures, we are establishing processes and associations that transmit values, and values that influence behavior.

We all know that self-esteem, responsibility, and faith are the essentials of strong communities and families. We must have them to be able to care for others, maintain relationships, give love. They provide the reserves that allow us to tolerate frustration, roll with the punches, contribute, create, hope, get up, and try again. It's the difference between the parent who wants to kill his kid for crying all night and the one who resists such evil.

What we hope for are organizations and associations that transmit such virtues as faith (gives hope), responsibility (that leads toward being obligated toward your family and community), discipline (that leads to working hard in self and others), and commitment (leading to cooperation and mutual accountability) so that in the end we will learn how to love our family and our neighbors.

Therefore, any strategy in a community must reinforce those organizations and associations that strengthen the ties that bind—that link habits of the heart with habits of the mind.

CONCLUSION

Something is going on beneath the surface. In spite of all the dreary demographics and rhetoric coming out of Washington, the stresses in our system have forced us to draw on hidden resources to create a new and better order—new modes of problem solving, new social entities, new ways of distributing power.

A corollary to Murphy's Law states, "Anything that goes wrong can be used to your advantage, provided it goes wrong enough." At first glance, that doesn't seem to make a lot of sense. But when you think about it in light of recent years that have been the worst possible times for social programs, it begins to mean something.

When there is a policy vacuum, a stagnation of the bureaucracy, gaps in the system arise. Those gaps can be filled by new energy and creative ideas. A system going wrong, getting disconnected, opens up voids. These voids are chances to permeate the old with the new. I think that's what we are seeing on the neighborhood level and in some corporations—the new social forms of partnership investment strategies and networking arising from the shell of the old ideologies.

The challenge for us today is to help people on the local level build the support systems for a technological society working in neighborhoods and communities. And we can help the poor help themselves to gain a sense of power and self-esteem in the process.

What I am trying to convey to you is that the role of caring and advocacy never ends. We must make a genuine, complete commitment of caring and advocacy both daylong and lifelong. We have to be prepared to use our professional skills and our internal values throughout our lives, not just when we're going to meetings. Our talents and skills can be of enormous help to the people in our own communities who are battling racism, sexism, and shrinking economic opportunity.

Together we will go forward to build communities, we will go on working to take care of the children, caring for the elderly, trying to keep the family whole and healthy. Although it may appear to be moving slowly, or not at all, I believe and I know that we can make changes for the better, and we will. Democracy is at stake.

REFERENCES

Borlias, G.J. (1992). Ethnic capital and intergeneration mobility. In *Quarterly Journal of Economics,* February 1992, 123-150.

Case, A. and Katz, S. (1992). *The Company You Keep: The Effects of Family and Neighborhood on Disadvantaged Youth.* Cambridge, MA: National Bureau of Economic Research, NBER Working Paper No. 3705.

Coleman, J.S. and Hoffer, T.B. (1987). *Public and Private High Schools: The Impact of Communities.* New York: Basic Books.

Comer, J. (1980). *School Power.* New York: The Free Press.

Connell, J., Kubisch, A., Schon, L., and Weiss, C. (1995). *New Approaches to Evaluation Community Initiatives: Concepts and Methods.* Washington, DC: The Aspen Institute.

Coulton, C. (1989). *An Analysis of Poverty and Related Conditions in Cleveland Area Neighborhoods.* Cleveland, OH: Case Western Reserve University.

Coyle, G.L. (1947). *Group Experience and Democratic Values*, p. 142. New York: Woman's Press.

Eisen, A. (1992). *Report on Foundations Collaboration with Comprehensive Neighborhood-Based Community Empowerment Initiatives.* New York Community Trust. Unpublished paper.

Ferguson, M. (1990). *The Aquarian Conspiracy: Personal and Social Transformations in the 1980s.* New York: J.P. Tarcher, Inc.

Garvin, C. and Cox, F. (1995). A history of community organizing since the Civil War with special reference to oppressed communities. In J.R. Rothman, J. Erlich, and J. Tropman (Eds.), *Strategies of Community Intervention.* Itasca, IL: F.E. Peacock, 64-98.

Kretzmann, J. and McKnight, J. (1993). *Building Communities from the Inside Out: A Path Toward Finding and Mobilizing Communities' Assets.* Evanston, IL: Northwestern University.

Melaville, A. and Blank, M. (1991). *What It Takes: Structuring Interagency Partnerships to Connect Children and Families with Comprehensive Services.* Washington, DC: Education and Human Services Consortium.

Naparstek, A., Biegel, D., and Spiro, H. (1982). *Neighborhood Networks for Human Mental Health Care.* New York: Plenum Press.

Palmer, J. and Sawhill, J. (1982). Perspective on the Reagan experiment. In J. Palmer and J. Sawhill (Eds.), *The Reagan Experiment: An Examination of Economic and Social Policies Under the Reagan Administration.* Washington, DC: Urban Institute, 15-19.

Putnam, R. (1993). *Making Democracy Work: Civic Traditions in Modern Italy.* Princeton, NJ: Princeton University Press.

Rubin, H. and Rubin, J. (1992). *Community Organization and Recruitment.* New York: Macmillan.

Spergal, J. (1972). *Community Organization and Development.* New York: Macmillan.

Svirdoff, M. (1994). The seeds of urban revival. *The Public Interest*, 114 (Winter), 82-103.

Walsh, J. (1996). *Stories of Renewal: Community Building and the Future of Urban America.* New York: Rockefeller Foundation.

Wilson, W.J. (1991). Public policy research and the truly disadvantaged. In C. Jencks and P. Peterson (Eds.), *The Urban Underclass*, pp. 460-482. Washington, DC: Brookings Institute.

Chapter 3

From the Local to the Global: Groups at the Heart of the Community

Audrey Mullender

(This presentation was preceded by an interchange of morning greetings in seventeen languages and dialects, and through nonverbal communication.)

There is an argument, currently, that the nation state is obsolete. Arthur C. Clarke pronounced recently, appropriately enough in an interview broadcast to the United Kingdom by satellite from his home in Asia, that the nation state is too big for the individual yet too small for the world. Despite the resurgence of nationalism in many parts of the globe, Clarke's view is that the communications revolution—together, one could also argue, with the role now played by multinational companies in the global economy and the need to preserve the environment—means that we must now conceptualize our lives on a worldwide scale and not as if confined to our own national corner. Of course, my own country thought of itself on a global scale once before, in the days of the British Empire, but that was about domination, whereas the new globalization needs to be about learning and sharing together if we are to survive into the twenty-first century.

If Clarke is right, we might say that we now live in our local village (which may be our own community or neighborhood within a town or city) and in the global village, with nothing much that makes sense in between. It is my contention that group work can help us to build communities, both at the most local level (something we have always done as group workers, from the settlements onward) and to unite the global village. Telephone groups (Regan, 1996) and networks on the World Wide Web have helped us to realize that people no longer need physically to meet together in order to form a group whose members can support one another through anger, pain, and joy. And people with a shared cause increasingly find ways to meet or communicate together on an ever-widening scale: women from every nation on earth at the conference in 1996 in Beijing in China, gay and lesbian people traveling from all over everywhere to San Francisco, or to Mardi Gras in Sydney, Australia, or to the lesbian tent at the Beijing women's conference; the international movement of disabled people; the diasporas of African, of Jewish, of Irish people who recognize common cause—all have something which means more to them than individualistic or nationalistic politics of self-interest.

In this sense, "global" is different from "international" because it refers to something over and above—outside of, and beyond—the concept of nations. In the same vein, travel around the globe becomes far more than tourism if we journey in order to learn and grow together, rather than to impose who we already are upon some fresh people. In view of this latter point, I want to qualify this and say that I believe this only works if we can combine a transcultural, transnational, generalizable base of group work knowledge, values, and skills with a sensitivity to the most localized expression of human communication and expression of human need. In other words, group work is not a polyglot dictionary that contains all the answers in all the languages for the global traveler. Rather, it is a passport which, used with discretion, can get us through many doors but, once over the threshold, we find ourselves guests in another culture where we have to use our group work antennae to listen and learn how things may work differently in this new place.

At the same time, cultural relativity must be combined with an overarching anti-oppressive awareness which tells us that (almost?) every nation and (almost?) every culture on earth oppresses women, gay men and lesbians, disabled people, often its oldest and youngest citizens, poor people, and all whose ethnic and/or religious grouping has not held the political power. So we need to attune ourselves to a many-stranded communication in each new place which gives an ear for what local women are saying, local disabled people, and so on. In other words, there is a dynamic of change in each community, in each nation, and globally, to which we also need to be sensitive and with which we have a responsibility to ally ourselves. We are not passive tourists who look out of the bus windows as we drive past, or through a camera lens as if at a *tableau vivant* arranged for our benefit, but travelers on a shared journey into an uncertain future where our very survival on this planet is threatened by pollution, war, and exploitation of every kind. The social work agenda of "anti-discriminatory" (Thompson, 1992) and "anti-oppressive practice" in the United Kingdom and of "diversity" and "empowerment" here in the United States, should, in my view, expand to incorporate an awareness of these environmental and global imperatives. Green politics, i.e., social and community activism on environmental issues, in community work (Lane, 1997, writing in Australia) is telling us that this is the same quest for safe, peaceful, and healthy co-existence as the move toward race, ability, age, class, and sexual (gender *and* sexual orientation) equality—not a different one.

To summarize thus far, then, we set forth already partly equipped for our travels because we are group workers. On top of this, we need to learn that all interaction has a cultural basis *and* that all interaction expresses a dynamic of power or powerlessness. Perhaps we might express one of the group worker's valid roles as that of "diplomat"—learning the interactional patterns of another way of life: the means, for example, of expressing comprehension, pleasure, anger, or distrust so as to be able to engage in effective intra- and intergroup communication and negotiation, but doing so within a context where some people hold more cards than others, and where some have more to lose because they are already living on the edge of survival. Our arrival into this context may be far from neutral.

So this diplomat must not only be good at languages, so as to interpret what he or she observes and hears on his or her travels, but equipped, too, with a set of principles which underpin the interpretation of all the new experiences and help make the decisions as to how and whether to intervene. The values of group work practice form a crucial basis for judging what forms and contexts of communication are likely to be appropriate and what power dynamics they convey. The principles I would wish to espouse (Mullender and Ward, 1991) stress, among other things: the abilities of all people, the oppressed as well as the dominant; the need for all those who intervene in other people's lives to engage in an active fight against oppression; and the view that the most helpful way to intervene is not as a pseudo "expert," but as someone who may perhaps facilitate others to find their own answers. I will return to these values later.

THE GLOBAL TRAVELER IN GROUP WORK— AN EXAMPLE

An experience which was most challenging to my skills as a group worker was one involving Maori participants in New Zealand—the other side of the world from the United Kingdom—where I had gone to spend a term's sabbatical. I had been engaged to run a two-day workshop in a town at the southern tip of the South Island. I arrived the day before to discover—too late to stop people from making quite long journeys to participate—that I, a "Pakeha" or person of white European descent, was assigned as a visiting "expert" to "teach" an entirely Maori group in the setting of a Maori agency. Not only did this cut across all the empowering principles of my approach (I do not seek to work as an expert teacher) but I was also plunged into an ethically unacceptable situation as a white person brought in to train a black group (i.e., a group of persons of color). How this had transpired was that the white agency who booked me had been full of poorly analyzed liberal goodwill and had wanted to share the "privilege" of my visit with those groups who normally had fewest formal training opportunities. Nevertheless, what they had set up was bound to create mistrust of their motives and to collude with assumptions that they and I believed in white Western superiority. Furthermore, at a practical level, I had only recently arrived and had the most rudimentary knowledge of the intricate and ritualized traditional Maori meeting structures, knew perhaps three words in the Maori language and—devastating for a group worker—soon discovered that I could not read the nonverbal cues or signals either from individuals or from the group. How could I survive?

What I did was to fall back on the value base which underpins all my practice, training, and research work and to look for ways to express those values nonverbally.

My work is built upon a particular set of practice principles contained in the book *Self-Directed Groupwork: Users Take Action for Empowerment* (Mullender and Ward, 1991). These were gathered through a practice-based research exercise that identified the key elements of the ways in which empowering group workers were operating. The principles are as follows:

1. We need to take a view of the people we work with which refuses to accept negative labels, and recognizes instead that all people have skills, understanding, and ability. (I needed to look for those abilities.)
2. People have rights, including the right to be heard, the right to choose what kinds of intervention to accept in their lives, and the right to define issues and take action on them. (I needed to emphasize those rights.)
3. The problems that service users face are complex and responses to them need to reflect this. People's problems can never be fully understood if they are seen solely as a result of personal inadequacies. Issues of oppression, social policy, and environment and the economy are, more often than not, major contributory forces. Practice should reflect this understanding. (I needed to make sure mine did.)
4. Practice can effectively be built on the knowledge that people acting collectively can be powerful. People who lack power can gain it through working together in groups. (I needed to help the group feel powerful.)
5. Methods of working must reflect nonelitist principles. Workers do not "lead" the group but facilitate members in making decisions for themselves and in controlling whatever outcome ensues. Though special skills and knowledge are employed, these do not accord privilege and are not solely the province of the workers. (I needed to be a facilitator, not a leader.)
6. All our work must challenge oppression—whether by reason of race, gender, sexual orientation, age, class, disability, or any other form of social differentiation upon which spurious no-

tions of superiority and inferiority are kept in place by the exercise of power. (I needed to be aware of my own power as a professional and as a white person, and to find anti-oppressive ways to work.)

These values were expressed, first of all, through my standing in the middle of the group, explaining the dilemma I faced, and physically tearing up the written agenda. I then handed over to the participants the right to construct their own use of time, with me as facilitator as required. This showed that I valued their own strengths and abilities and did not regard myself as having spurious expertise over them. They quickly taught me, for example, that written materials are not trusted because they belong to the white, Western tradition, not to the largely oral Maori tradition. (New Zealand is, most notably, still untangling the implications of the written-down Treaty of Waitangi, not least because the white signatories believed it was possible to own land while the Maori people believe it is only possible to exercise stewardship over it; furthermore, that those who are "of the land," the *"tangata whenua,"* will always, inalienably be so. These differences of perspective will no doubt resonate with native and immigrant American people.)

After this, a day of testing my motives, my sincerity and what I had to offer was followed by a day of intense and fruitful work and future planning, based on more appropriate foundations. The value base I espoused turned out to provide important common ground between the participants and myself. Literally seating myself, at one point, at the feet of a Maori community leader, to listen quietly to his words when he rose to speak, I certainly learned as much as I gave—and I won respect by showing it. I and the group came out of this experience mutually enriched, but only because of the values we shared. We used them to find a way to communicate. At the end, I was made the most spiritually significant gift in Maori terms, of greenstone jewelry. (Some years later, this was stolen from my home in the United Kingdom in a burglary—in a region of the country where all the traditional trades of ship building, mining, and so on have been systematically destroyed by a government that fears to hear the voice of organized labor and favors cheap imports from countries where the workforce is employed on starvation wages, a region where many have felt that turning to dishonesty was the only way to feed their families. I have often wondered what impact that greenstone has had in someone else's life because traditionally it conveys ill luck if purchased for money—I am not sure what is thought to happen if it is stolen!)

Thinking back to that experience in New Zealand, at the end of the first day, I was in despair and close to tears, so little nonverbal feedback did I seem to be getting. On the second morning, I asked a woman, senior in years, why there was so little sign of participation. Her reply was simple: "I have come back. I am here." It seems that her traditional, nonverbal sign of discontent would simply have been to leave and that what, to me, looked like stony faced nonreceptiveness was a respectful, attentive listening. I had looked at the surface instead of into the heart.

After this experience, and others in New Zealand, I reflected how many group work techniques are an artificial Western replacement for what our communities, wherever they are, once knew instinctively. This is why deep-seated cultures, such as the Maori and the Native American, are so fascinating for group workers. While we have struggled to reinvent exercises to break the ice with people from whom our societies alienate us (as we live in our consumer bubbles), cultures we have oppressed have been refinding and revaluing traditional ways of coming together to share experiences and solve problems in groups. On the very day that I was word processing this chapter, an item on the news in the United Kingdom reported that Maori family group meeting structures are being translated on an experimental basis into some juvenile justice practice in the United Kingdom, as they have already been into work to find solutions for children whose families need support (Family Rights Group, 1994). Those local groups now have global significance in teaching us how to live together in mutual support rather than mutual mistrust and destruction.

It strikes me forcibly that the struggles of the so-called developed world to invent exercises for ice breaking, exercises for warm-ups, exercises to enhance participation, are perhaps only needed because we have lost so much of our traditional ability to coexist naturally, to express ourselves and to overcome our inevitable human dilemmas in groups. Maori people, similar to Native American people and others all over the globe, are working hard to discover their ability to do this after a history of white oppression which sought to destroy their language, their culture, their identity. Maori meeting structures—now used for conferences, teaching, and every kind of public gathering—have group-based introductions moving from the women's welcome to the *marae* (the meeting place) and the men's war dancing, through ritualized greetings, to the more intimate "round robin" of personal introductions and then of encircling and nose touching (or handshaking if Western inhibitions persist). At all times, the relationship between the group of hosts and the group of visitors is visible as it progresses through the stages of challenge, testing out, acceptance and, finally, respect and friendship. This is a marvelous, and salutory experience for any group worker—to see a group work process which has traversed many centuries and which is as relevant now for a workshop on child abuse as it is for a religious ceremony. In Auckland, there is even a social work program that operates its classroom along Maori lines, with shoes left at the door, songs and greetings to start the day, and traditionally respectful ways of listening to one another's ideas.

ASKING THE QUESTION, "WHY?"

In Maori gatherings, I found the values I outlined earlier to be very much in evidence, including a seeking after social change to right the wrongs of the past. Some group workers have taken the view that these values amount to nothing more than common sense and basic good practice, and that they are already putting them into practice. When one analyzes their work in more depth, however, the one value of the six that is most commonly forgotten is the third—problems are complex and not the result of personal inadequacy—and yet, what we most need to learn to do on a global scale is to activate that third value of self-directed group work, the one which stresses the social structural complexity of the problems people face. Working with group members to analyze WHY the issues they have identified exist is the distinctive feature of practice which seeks to achieve empowerment. Without it, there can be no awareness of wider-scale oppression, no moving beyond people blaming themselves for their problems (or believing it when other people do so; cf. Ryan, 1971) into greater awareness and the pursuit of social change. To jump straight from identifying WHAT is wrong into the practicalities (the HOW) of achieving change, as so often happens, is to collude with a process in which explanations of the responsibility for problems are usually sought in the private world around individual and family, either because this is the extent of the worker's own understanding or because it appears to them to make intervention more feasible. To ask the question WHY?, on the other hand, brings social issues into play and opens up new options for action in the public world. It represents the application of the values of resistance and empowerment in practice. These values are as important globally as they are locally.

Indeed, the techniques for asking Why have historically spread from one people to another around the globe. Paulo Freire's (1972) conscientization work with Brazilian peasants, for example, has influenced self-directed group work in the United Kingdom (Mullender and Ward, 1991), Lee's (1994) empowerment model, the work of Gutierrez and her colleagues with Latino populations here in the United States (e.g., Gutierrez and Ortega, 1991), and the writing of Margot Breton (1994, 1995) in Canada. Breton (1992) has also drawn upon Latin American liberation theology to offer important lessons for group work with oppressed people. Looking further back, the technique of "speaking bitterness"—sitting in a circle and speaking in turn about the everyday circumstances and events of life, with no one remaining silent, no one interrupting or passing comment—spread from China to the early women's consciousness-raising groups in the United States and, from there, around the world. Just as the peasants in China "were able to change their lives by examining their own personal everyday experience of oppression . . . [getting] a lot of strength from talking about it and comparing stories" (Alix Kates Shulman, 1979, pp. 228-229), so did the women in those early groups. These techniques made it possible to share things which would have seemed inconsequential or wrong-headed in other circumstances—in circumstances where women are silenced by men, for example, where poor people are expected to defer to the wealthy and powerful, and, I would stress, wherever group members are told what to do by group workers.

Women, Brazilian and Chinese peasants, disability equality activists, and many others have slowly learned to recognize and to value their own and one another's experiences and, in turn, to voice these more freely. Gradually, it has emerged, for example, that women around the world have in common the same feelings of drudgery, duty, guilt, implied inadequacy, anger, and fear. Issues that individuals had not previously even recognized as such—e.g., who performed basic chores in the home, or how men assumed they had a right to control women—were heard repeatedly until the conclusion became inescapable that they affected all women, from all backgrounds, *and could not be attributable any longer to individual failings on the part of those women.* It was the fundamental relationships between men and women, and women's own valuation of themselves, as well as society's valuation of them, which needed to change. There are exact parallels for every other oppressed group.

The upshot of this is that it is not the victim but the oppression which is the problem, that we need less therapy and more social action—and that this is certainly true in respect of many of the most widespread problems in our communities. Through that social action, individuals will also learn how to grow and change.

Staying with my example of the women's movement, we have more recently moved on to a recognition that women's rights are human rights (Bunch and Carrillo, 1992). The UN and the World Bank are concerning themselves with women's issues, not because their policymakers have suddenly all become feminists, but because they are recognizing that women's safety and women's education will have the most effective impact on the future of the globe and of the global economy. The women's meeting in Beijing last year already knew this. The national representatives who gather in Geneva, in New York, in Brussels (for the European Union), in Pan-African and Asian-Pacific gatherings, need to learn these things too. And, once again, there are exact parallels for every oppressed group, as, for example, a civil and human rights model is adopted by disabled people to fight for access to jobs and services, drawing directly from the civil rights movement among African Americans.

The raised awareness of the black consciousness movement in the United States affords an interesting example of a spread into social work at a local level. It worked on confronting and reversing the negative valuation of dominant white society and, in its early days, adopted the slogan "Black is beautiful." It is exciting to see this raised awareness working through into social work and into group work. In Manchester, England, a group of young black people in care called the "Black and In Care Group" produced a newsletter which took *Black Is Beautiful* as its title and linked broader international awareness of landmark events in black oppression (such as the continuing imprisonment and, later, the release of Nelson Mandela) with the need for a detailed analysis of the way black children are treated in the white care system: whether ethnic food is cooked, whether black history and culture are celebrated, whether racist language is outlawed, and whether aware black families are found to foster and adopt black children. Those young people were giving us a perfect example of how global awareness and local awareness can be combined, and of how a historically overlooked and oppressed group can build its own sense of direction, of influence, and of a community of interest through resisting oppression.

INTERVENTION FOR RESISTANCE AGAINST OPPRESSION

The workers' role in this What and Why work is to see that topics emerge from the group and are kept in play long enough for the necessary broader understanding—the "why" to develop. Hope and Timmel (1984, p. 60), writing in an African context, summarize the prompts for the ensuing discussion as a series of questions (adapted slightly here):

1. Description—*What do you see happening?*
2. Analysis—*Why is it happening?*
3. Related problems—*What problems does it lead to?*
4. Root Causes—*What are the root causes of these problems?*
5. Action planning—*What can we do about it?*

Mullender and Ward (1991) have summarized this same series of questions as What?, Why?, and How?. Since the Why is the one most frequently ignored, it is useful to look at a technique, utilized on a global scale, which has been developed to give it full prominence.

Ah-Hah! Seminars

A full-scale technique for undertaking this work is that of the Ah-Hah! Seminar (GATT-Fly, 1983), developed by a Canadian project to work with popular groups, including native people's organizations around the globe for economic justice. The "popular education" methodology involves asking participants to create a pictorial representation of their world, showing the interrelationships of the different features in it, so that they understand clearly for the first time what they knew before in only a partial or confused way (hence the title of the seminars). It makes the link from the local to the global.

Those present at an Ah-Hah! Seminar sit in a semicircle around a large sheet of paper, with colored felt pens available to draw symbols representing various aspects of their lives and the life of their community. Participants can ask one another questions about their drawings and the facilitator also prompts people to think about different parts of their lives and how they fit together, as well as valuing contributions as they are added. In particular, participants may need encouraging to do the first drawings. These start with a symbol central to the particular group or the reason for holding the seminar: for example, a women's group put a feminist activist at the heart of its drawing while a group of Native Americans discussing day care put their children at the center. Although the facilitator can also join in, he or she should not start the drawing off since this can hold others back. It also helps if earlier work in the group has included drawing. Nothing elaborate is needed; stick people are perfectly adequate, especially as the drawings are discussed as the work goes along.

People are asked to name the symbols they are drawing and to explain their significance. The facilitator ensures that plenty of time is devoted to this. Probing questions are asked about each element of the picture: "What is she doing, this feminist activist? Whose interests does she serve? Who needs her? What problems does she address? What are the factors influencing this situation? What else is going on? How are these factors connected to each other?" (Adams, undated, p. 5). In particular, the prevailing political, economic, and social forces are analyzed in detail: "Who benefits from the status quo, who loses out, and in what ways? How do all these things link up?" On this analysis, more effective action for change will later be based.

The result of the exercise is that people are enabled to build a picture of the wider social system, on a local, national, or global scale (or all three), focused around their own place in it. They can then discuss how it is maintained in this form, what needs to change (all linked up in one color), and what can be done to achieve this. The strengths of the model are its simplicity as a technique, the complexity and interrelatedness of the resulting analysis, the graphic and comprehensible form in which this emerges, the affirmation that groups can conduct their own structural analysis, and the added benefits of developing group control over process and offering an entertaining and creative way of learning.

This technique is cooperative and hence helps people to arrive at a collective analysis of their own situation. There is often a low point during the session (which ideally requires a day or two to do properly) when participants see how many powerful forces they have portrayed, all of which are ranged against them (Adams, undated, p. 3). With facilitation, however, this can also be the turning point, before the second half of the discussion time turns toward making plans for action. The facilitator tries to ensure that resources and strengths have been included in the picture before this stage in addition to all the problems: features such as networks, friends, allies, people's own strengths and motivations, past successes of the group, other individuals and groups affected by the same negative social forces, and so on, can all be called on when it comes to planning how to fight back. The facilitator needs group process skills, perhaps shared with the group, not only to read the overall emotional climate, but also to encourage the group to look at any blocks which occur and to deal with apparently contradictory views.

A version of the Ah-Hah! technique was used as a full-day workshop at a women's conference. It had to be "consistent with the feminist principles that the personal is political, and that women's perspective should be central to our work for social change" (Lewis, 1988, p. 1). The facilitators helped the group to start from women's family and home lives, and then to draw in work, community, and the work of women's groups in the region. The wall-sized "maps" of women's lives which resulted were a graphic representation of the complexity of women's experience. Later, the participants "analyzed the results by looking for the connections between our lives and the social and political institutions that shape much of our experience. We asked who has control over the problems women face, and who benefits. Finally, we asked ourselves what changes would result in real improvements in our lives" (Lewis, 1988, p. 1). Examples of answers to this question were: flexible child care arrangements and work schedules, services planned and controlled by the communities they serve, equality of access to education and expansion of job training for women, and events which are made accessible to isolated, low income, disabled, black, and Native American women. They found this way of working to be an empowering technique which, because it pushes participants toward seeking their own solutions, has the advantage of offering a natural progression into continuing work.

The technique has been used all over the world. In Malaysia, a female rubber plantation worker recognized the links between her own situation and that of electronics workers in her country who needed to become unionized, while a participant at a seminar in Thailand stated that:

> . . . participants . . . feel they are active, rather than responsive. As a result, they realize their power that they can make the whole world [change]; they can dictate to the world; and they realize what potential they have. (Howlett, 1985, p. 2)

Similar challenges to recognize and change the local world in a way which also makes sense for the globe are present in the starkest form all over Eastern Europe, the Middle East—and in our national backyards.

CONCLUSION

My Symposium hosts' nation and mine have exported many things around the globe in the past—cultural imperialism, the English language, Coca-Cola, running shoes, McDonald's, popular music. The fact that I can go to the other side of the globe from my home and see the same queen portrayed on the banknotes when I arrive, speak the same language at every port of call, and even drive on the left for the whole trip (if I don't make too many stops) tells me that there is a history to thinking on a global level.

Up to now, though, this has mainly happened at the expense of those communities which used to flourish locally. It is my belief that there are principles within the group work canon, and skills belonging to all group workers, which could actually help us both to rebuild locally *and* to cooperate globally. The damage we have inflicted on our planet and its peoples is vast. Can our work for change be pursued with anything like the same vigor that wreaked the destruction? We will need to combine energy with humility, the offer of assistance with the ability to listen, the skill to intervene with the patience to comprehend diversity and complex power dynamics. Good group workers have these combinations of skills and values. Both the knowledge base and the practice base need to be developed in ways which accord them the first place.

Coda

But a note of caution. Groups can be powerful for harm as well as good. Pedophile rings, the Ku Klux Klan, the Nuremberg rallies, those committees of the great and the good who decide that gay and lesbian people are not fit to foster or adopt, or that disabled people need segregated schooling, all employ the structure and process of groups to visit their outright or their well-meaning damage upon the world. Coming together as a group merely creates undirected energy. It is the values we choose to apply which give that energy direction. The challenge to group workers is to choose their principles as carefully as they hone their skills, to analyze their impact on prevailing power dynamics as clearly as they explore intragroup dynamics, to ask the local and the global question Why? as well as the immediately practice-oriented questions What? and How?

With all those things in place, we perhaps can begin to place groups at the heart of the local and the global community and to work for a more principled form of change. And, incidentally, the six principles and the question Why? could also be used by AASWG in some very interesting ways to think its way forward into becoming a more inclusive organization.

REFERENCES

Adams, J. (undated). *Ah-Hah! Seminar!!!*, Toronto, Ontario, Canada: Unpublished leaflet.

Breton, M. (1992). Liberation theology, group work, and the right of the poor and oppressed to participate in the life of the community, *Social Work with Groups, 15*(2/3), pp. 257-269.

Breton, M. (1994). On the meaning of empowerment and empowerment-oriented social work practice, *Social Work with Groups, 17*(3), pp. 23-37.

Breton, M. (1995). The potential for social action in groups, *Social Work with Groups, 18*(2/3), pp. 5-13.

Bunch, C. and Carrillo, R. (1992). *Gender Violence: A Development and Human Rights Issue*, Dublin, Ireland: Attic Press.

Family Rights Group (1994). *Family Group Conferences*, London: Family Rights Group.

Freire, P. (1972). *Pedagogy of the Oppressed*, Harmondsworth, UK: Penguin.

GATT-Fly (1983). *Ah-Hah! A New Approach to Popular Education*, Toronto, Ontario, Canada: Between the Lines Press.

Gutierrez, L.M. and Ortega, R. (1991). Developing methods to empower Latinos: The importance of groups, *Social Work with Groups, 14*(2), pp. 23-43.

Hope, A. and Timmel, S. (1984). *Training for Transformation.* Gweru, Zimbabwe: Mambo Press.

Howlett, D. (1985). Asian Ah-Hahs, *GATT-Fly Report: A Periodical on Global Issues of Economic Justice*, November, *VI* (3), pp. 1-3.

Lane, M. (1997). Community work, social work: Green and postmodern, *British Journal of Social Work, 27*(3), pp. 319-341.

Lee, J.A.B. (1994). *The Empowerment Approach to Social Work Practice*, New York: Columbia University Press.

Lewis, D.J. (1988). *Putting Women on the Map: Building an Agenda for Change*, Vancouver, B.C., Canada: Women's Research Centre [Leaflet].

Mullender, A. and Ward, D. (1991). *Self-Directed Groupwork: Users Take Action for Empowerment*, London: Whiting and Birch.

Regan, S. (1996). Teleconferencing: Group counseling and the theme-centered interactional model. Paper presented at the European Group Work Symposium, "Groups at the Heart of Working with People," Bournemouth, UK, July 17-19, 1996.

Ryan, W. (1971). *Blaming the Victim*, New York: Pantheon.

Shulman, A.K. (1979). *Burning Questions*, London: André Deutsch.

Thompson, N. (1992). *Anti-Discriminatory Practice*, Basingstoke, UK: Macmillan.

SECTION II:
INVITATIONALS

Chapter 4

Toward a Community of Care: The Development of the Family Caregivers' Support Network

Jennifer Poole

The plight of the family caregiver has been well documented. We know that most senior care in the community is provided by a family member. We know these family members are usually wives, daughters, or other female relatives, and we know what the financial, emotional, and physical costs of family care can be for both the caregiver and the care receiver (Fradkin and Liberti, 1994).

To alleviate this burden, various educational and mutual support programs have been implemented to provide technical, social, and emotional support for the family/informal caregiver. Few programs, however, are facilitated by the caregivers themselves, and few programs are on their way to becoming freestanding and self-sufficient communities of caregivers advocating, networking, and supporting each other. This chapter reports on the progress of one such community in the making, a program in progress called the Family Caregivers Support Network, based in Toronto, Canada.

WHAT IS CAREGIVING?

It has been suggested that researchers and practitioners have only a vague notion of what caregiving really is (Barer and Johnson, 1990). The term has been used to describe a wide variety of primary and secondary functions including homemaking, housing, income, support, personal care, home health care, transportation, psychological support, social and recreational activities, spiritual support, protection and bureaucratic mediation (Barer and Johnson, 1990). Researchers have also chronicled the *stages* in the careers of a family caregiver from residential caregiving to institutional placement and bereavement (Pearlin, 1992). Rather than simply a function, caregiving is more a process driven by changing demands and contexts, activities and dispositions (Pearlin, 1992).

The caregivers involved with the project I present today define themselves as individuals who look after and or/advocate for an elderly person. The ways, means, and locations of that care will, and often do, vary.

WHO ARE THE CAREGIVERS?

At present, social policy in Canada is influenced by an atmosphere of fiscal panic (Bornstein, 1994). Like an expensive "hot potato," care of the elderly has been passed by the federal government to the provincial government and then to the community (Bornstein, 1994). Publicly funded health and social services account for only 10 to 15 percent of the total care of the elderly in Canada (Aronson, 1992). The rest is provided by the family, and family care is often a euphemism for the care provided by women (Aronson, 1992; Guberman, Maheu, and Maille, 1992; Hartman, 1990).

The reliance on women as caregivers of the elderly does not mean that men are absent from informal helping networks. Husbands and wives frequently reallocate household chores to cope with infirmity, and as my eighty-five-year-old grandfather has demonstrated, husbands do provide excellent personal and health care for their frail spouses (Stoller, 1990). However, research suggests that the contributions of sons and other male helpers may be more limited in terms of time, range, and intensity (Stoller, 1990). Men may help with occasional tasks such as shopping, financial management, and heavy chores but are less likely to assist with routine chores such as the dishes, personal care, and laundry (Stoller, 1990).

WHY CARE?

Various researchers have attempted to answer the question, why do women often provide "family" care for the elderly? Documented reasons include feelings of love and duty, family ties, inadequacy of community resources, a need to help others, imposition of the decision, women's economic dependence, family tradition, and the unavailability of other family members (Guberman, Maheu, and Maille, 1992). Other findings have suggested that lower socioeconomic class (Rosenthal and Gladstone, 1994) and ethnicity (Sokolovsky, 1991) affect a woman's decision to provide care to her aging kin. Distrust of professional care may also prompt a family caregiver to decline or ration the amount of support she seeks from the "community," further intensifying the burdens of her caregiving (Aronson, 1992).

For some, there are some very positive benefits of family caregiving such as being able to keep the care receiver at home (Cohen et al., 1994). However, a majority of caregivers may experience many of the more negative aspects of caregiving, including emotional and financial pressures, inconvenience, anxiety, and depression (Biegel, Shore, and Gordon, 1984). Besides the emotional and financial strain and the drain on her own family and social life, a woman caregiver who also leaves her job to care for her aging kin must "consider the lost opportunities to accumulate pension benefits or equity" (Aronson, 1989, p. 118). In this way, a woman's decision not to work outside the home in order to care for an elderly relative is often a prelude to poverty in old age (Aronson, 1989).

SOCIAL PROGRAMS AND SUPPORTS
FOR CAREGIVERS

To lessen the burden placed on family caregivers and assist them in their role, various family caregiver "enhancement" strategies have been developed over the past twenty years. However, there is neither agreement nor conclusive evidence as to which strategy is the most effective in reducing the caregiving burden (Whitlatch, Zarit, and Von Eye, 1991). Others charge that "enhancement" strategies only further disempower caregivers, for they assume rather than question that the family or, rather, women will automatically provide care (Aronson, 1992).

Biegel, Shore, and Gordon (1984) classify these caregiver enhancement strategies into the following: (1) education and training programs (2) formalization and coordination programs and (3) mutual aid/self-help group strategies. The most common and easily implemented education and training programs aim to reduce stress by improving caregivers' technical skills and increasing caregivers' knowledge and understanding of issues associated with the aging process. These types of programs may involve a time-limited series of workshops on stress or patient care and the use of printed materials such as pamphlets, manuals, or other resources (Biegel, Shore, and Gordon, 1984). These programs are usually facilitated by a professional for a fee.

Formalization and coordination strategies aim to develop an overall service plan for the care receiver. The service package, developed by a professional facilitator and the family caregiver, details both informal and formal services to be used and may involve paying family caregivers for their service (Biegel, Shore, and Gordon, 1984). The strategy has been successfully implemented in the states of New York, Maine, and Kentucky.

Mutual aid and self-help groups assume that caregivers possess the necessary expertise and hold the solutions to many of their own problems (Biegel, Shore, and Gordon, 1984). Groups aim to reduce isolation, provide caregivers with support and hope, and improve problem-solving skills (Lavoie, 1995). Some groups are permanent, some temporary, some open to new members and some closed, some led by peers, and some co-led by professionals. Three types of groups have been identified in the literature; groups that focus on education, groups that focus on education and mutual support, and "ventilation groups" for people to express their feelings (Lavoie, 1995). For our purposes, we define a self-help group as a voluntary peer-led group of people who share a common problem or life experience such as family caregiving.

One review of the literature on the effectiveness of support groups for caregivers concluded that they "don't work" (Lavoie, 1995). However, this body of research was mostly limited to studies of short-term professionally led support groups which lend themselves more easily to pre- and post-test measures. Moreover, expectations that caregivers can improve their coping skills and depression by means of three of four workshops or group meetings may be unrealistic (Lavoie, 1995, p. 589). Very little research has been done on long-term, peer-led, self-help groups for caregivers, nor does the existing literature suggest we know what family caregivers really want. This is where the Family Caregivers' Support Network begins.

HISTORY OF THE FAMILY CAREGIVERS SUPPORT NETWORK AT THE SELF-HELP RESOURCE CENTRE

The Family Caregivers Support Network is at the end of the first of three years of federal Seniors Independence Program funding. This program in process is sponsored by the Self-Help Resource Centre of Greater Toronto, a nonprofit organization which promotes self-help and mutual aid groups and activities.

During the early stages of project planning (1989), committee members identified gaps in service for caregivers and a need for information sharing, advocacy, and support. Citing their own experiences with caregiving (both professionally and in the home) a sense of isolation and a desire for a more representative coordinating body, the group developed a proposal for a caregivers' network, focusing on peer support, mutual aid, information sharing and skill development (a combination of existing caregiver "enhancement" strategies). The Self-Help Resource Centre, which promotes self-help and mutual aid activities while providing educational and networking opportunities, seemed to be the natural home for the project.

The group then set five main goals for the new network:

1. Enable caregivers to maintain their dignity and independence
2. Encourage the development of self-help groups for caregivers of seniors
3. Empower a representative group of caregivers to advocate for other caregivers
4. Provide an information, referral, and support service for caregivers

5. Provide technical support and training for organizations which assist individuals caring for senior relatives or friends at home, in the community, in alternative residential arrangements, or acute and long-term institutional settings

To meet these goals, the group focused on implementing some of the activities which they felt were missing from community support programs for caregivers in Toronto. These activities included:

- Providing technical assistance to developing self-help groups for caregivers.
- Creating a database of community resources, supports, and self-help groups for caregivers.
- Developing an information and referral service.
- Publishing and distributing a newsletter.
- Providing training and educational workshops on issues identified by *caregivers.*
- Developing a peer support phone line staffed by caregivers for caregivers.
- Developing a caregiver-driven network structure which could begin to advocate, educate, and raise awareness about the caregiving process in Toronto and across Ontario.

BARRIERS TO FUNDING

The initial idea for the network was developed by 1989, but funding was not secured until 1995. This six-year funding process was fraught with difficulties, some of which were illustrated through participation in a "storytelling" project sponsored by the Centre for Health Promotion at the University of Toronto in December of 1994. The storytelling method uses structured dialogue to evaluate barriers to effective health promotion practice (Feather and Labonte, 1995). By first *describing* the barriers, then *explaining and reflecting* on them as a group, participants move toward a plan of action. Storytelling illustrated that as the issue of caregiver support became increasingly political, the proposal was passed like a "hot potato" from ministry to ministry. It also identified misconceptions about the role of self-help with seniors as a major obstacle to funding. Six rewrites, countless additions, and a few budget cuts later, the project was finally funded in the spring of 1995, three months after the storytelling workshop illustrated the obstacles between what the caregivers wanted to do and the means by which they could do it.

OUTCOMES OF THE PROJECT TO DATE

Although I call them outcomes, we have not used pre- and post-test measures for our "midterm report card." Instead, we have followed more of an implementation evaluation, looking at the process of setting up the network, the feelings of the participants, and the levels of participation by caregivers in all aspects of the network.

Methods including questionnaires, interviews, contact sheets, and storytelling have helped us to chart our progress so far and determine where the challenges are for the future of the project. In one short year, the work of the staff, volunteers, and advisory committee (all caregivers or former caregivers) has resulted in project outcomes listed below:

1. Implementation of an information and referral service for caregivers
2. Development of eight new self-help groups for caregivers
3. Development of a database of community resources for caregivers
4. Publication and distribution of four editions of the newsletter
5. Implementation of seven educational workshops for caregivers
6. Introduction of a new caregiver support telephone line
7. Recruitment of caregiver peer supporters
8. Development of a caregiver-driven network structure
9. Implementation of new outreach, research, and advocacy initiatives
10. Development of new mutual aid group for professional caregivers and professionals who work with caregivers

IMPLEMENTATION OF AN INFORMATION
AND REFERRAL SERVICE FOR CAREGIVERS

In its first year of operation, the Family Caregivers' Support Network has set up a fully operational information and referral service. Assistance is provided by staff and volunteers of the Family Caregivers' Support Network office in consultation with the project advisory committee. A number of important trends in this information and referral activity have been captured thus far:

- Requests for assistance have increased by more than 300 percent since the start of the project in 1995.
- Requests from professionals have increased by 400 percent.
- More caregivers are requesting assistance for the first time (60 percent).
- Most callers are asking for practical and emotional support (70 percent).

Contact sheets, completed for each call, suggest that most caregivers report hearing about the network through newspapers, TV spots, community agencies, word of mouth, and professionals.

DEVELOPMENT OF NEW SELF-HELP GROUPS
FOR CAREGIVERS

The community response to available support in developing new self-help/mutual aid options for caregivers has been overwhelming. Family Caregivers' Support Network staff have provided resources, consultation, technical assistance, as well as practical and emotional support to eight developing and "transitioning" self-help/mutual aid groups for caregivers. ("Transitioning" groups are those moving from professionally led to a peer-led group model.)

Assistance for these groups was provided by the Family Caregivers' Support Network after a request from a group member or a referring professional. These developing and transitioning groups provide the support to:

- Portuguese-speaking senior caregivers
- Caregivers serviced by an organization for seniors

• Rural caregivers in Northern Ontario
• Tamil caregivers in central Toronto
• Caregivers of patients at a Jewish long-term care facility
• Caregivers of elderly Holocaust survivors
• Caregivers dealing with depression
• Senior caregivers of dually diagnosed adults (both physically and mentally disabled)

DEVELOPMENT OF A DATABASE
OF COMMUNITY RESOURCES FOR CAREGIVERS

In addition to assisting new and developing groups for caregivers, the Family Caregivers' Support Network also provides caregivers with the only central listing of support groups in Toronto. The Family Caregivers' Support Network now lists over thirty-four groups for caregivers on its database. The majority of these groups (twenty-eight) are self-help/mutual aid groups, several are professionally led, and others are in varying stages of transition from professional to peer-led.

All groups are listed in the 1996 *Family Caregivers' Support Network Resource Directory*, produced by Family Caregivers' Support Network and available to any family caregiver free of charge. Directories are also made available to caregivers and professionals at all outreach events, displays, meetings, and conferences attended by Family Caregivers' Support Network staff as well as by request. To date, over 100 of these directories have been distributed to caregivers and health care workers, home care workers, and community outreach workers working with caregivers.

PUBLICATION AND DISTRIBUTION
OF A NEWSLETTER FOR CAREGIVERS

The Family Caregivers' Support Network has published four editions of the *Caregiving Network News*, and three more are planned for 1996. The current mailing list numbers approximately 2,000 contacts. Newsletters are also regularly distributed by various organizations in the community including Homecare, the Ontario Gerontology Association, the Alzheimer Society, long-term care facilities, resource centers across the city and the Self-Help Resource Centre. The Family Caregivers' Support Network also receives daily requests for additional copies and annual free subscriptions.

From the beginning, caregivers have been involved at all levels of production including writing, promotion, and consultation. Regular features address key issues identified by caregivers at the start of the project and through readership polls. These features include:

- New self-help groups in the community
- New community resources for caregivers
- Up-and-coming workshops
- Ways of taking care of oneself as a caregiver
- Stories of struggle and survival
- Cartoons, poems, and personal stories

According to one very isolated caregiver, the newsletter has also become a vital peer support tool, linking her with fellow caregivers across Toronto and surrounding areas. To that end, newsletter personnel are now in the process of adding a pen-pal section which will connect caregivers with other caregivers for mutual support, information, and friendship, especially when going to a meeting or a workshop is impossible or undesirable.

EDUCATIONAL WORKSHOPS FOR CAREGIVERS

Early in project development, caregivers identified accessible, affordable education and training workshops as vital practical supports. In response, the Family Caregivers' Support Network has held seven free workshops for caregivers, providing subsidies for transportation and respite care. Topics have included:

- Coping with Losses
- Improving Your Relationship with Professionals
- Relieving Stress
- Dealing with Anger and Guilt in Healthy Ways
- Humoring Yourself

- Tai Chi
- Relaxation

Caregivers response to the workshop series has been positive, with an average number of twenty participants at each workshop. Workshop evaluations provide planners with suggestions for scheduling and future topics. Some caregivers' comments on the workshops are listed below:

- I just wish I had been aware of this type of group one year ago. I feel I would have had an easier time.
- It felt great to walk into a group with many likeminded individuals. It was also very comforting.
- The main advantage was that we (members of a self-help group for caregivers) learned there is a way out of the rut we get ourselves into by getting stressed out and by letting stress rule us. These are good tools to take with us.
- Recognizing and dealing with anger is a large part of my caregiving. Thank you.

DEVELOPMENT OF A PEER SUPPORT SERVICE FOR CAREGIVERS

In addition to the peer support already actively taking place through publication and distribution of the newsletter, between participants at the workshops, between caregivers at the advisory meetings, and in developing and transitioning self-help groups, Family Caregivers' Support Network staff are implementing a peer support line staffed by caregivers for caregivers. The support line was designed by the initial project-planning group of caregivers to fill a gap in community support. Since that time, caregivers attending the workshops, in developing self-help groups, and those requesting assistance and support have reported that the line is "the most important part of Family Caregivers' Support Network because there is nothing else like it in Metro Toronto."

Colantonio, Cohen, and Corlett (1996) recently reported preliminary findings which support this approach. Their Seniors Independence Research Project-funded study on the "Support Needs of Family Caregivers" investigates the use of self-help and mutual-aid activities by older adults who are caregivers of persons with dementia. After asking caregivers what they would like to use in terms of self-help/mutual-aid services, it is "striking that the greatest demand for mutual aid was in the form of telephone support" (Colantonio, Cohen, and Corlett, 1996, p. 4). When leaving the house is not practical or possible, calling another caregiver for support becomes a significant and accessible form of support.

DEVELOPMENT OF A CAREGIVER-DRIVEN NETWORK STRUCTURE

In one year, the Family Caregivers' Support Network has also developed a strong foundation for an inclusive network structure. Upon the receipt of Senior Independence Program (SIP) funds from Health Canada, the advisory committee was formed with majority caregiver representation to direct and advise on all project activities and strategic planning. The committee is composed of representatives from caregivers' self-help groups, individual family caregivers, professional caregivers, former family caregivers, and project staff (both of whom are former family caregivers). This diversity of background, experience, knowledge, and involvement in caregiver support makes the committee viable, vital, and inclusive. Planning is about to begin in earnest to mount a campaign to develop a sustainable organizational structure, which is intended to be fully operational by the end of year three.

IMPLEMENTATION OF NEW OUTREACH, RESEARCH, AND ADVOCACY INITIATIVES FOR CAREGIVERS

To raise awareness about caregiving issues and the support available through the Family Caregivers' Support Network, members of the advisory committee and project staff have been actively networking, collaborating, and developing working relationships with government and sister groups and agencies that service caregivers.

Staff and volunteers have participated in over fifty local fairs and displays, conferences, symposia, and media events to raise awareness of the project and caregiving issues, including the World Health Organization/Centre for Health Promotion Summer Symposium 1996. Staff of the Family Caregivers' Support Network have also met with over thirty "sister" agencies supporting caregivers, accessing many of the professional support staff who work with more isolated family caregivers, and raising awareness about the potential role of self-help with this population.

In addition to this work, staff/advisory committee members have also been asked to provide consultation and a voice for caregivers on a number of new initiatives, including a carers' conference and the design and implementation of a new multicultural home day care service. The Family Caregivers' Support Network has also provided consultation to the Canadian Mental Health Association in designing a program to enhance and maintain existing peer support networks of caregivers for individuals with mental illness.

In terms of research, the Family Caregivers' Support Network has worked with a number of researchers exploring caregiving issues in Canada, notably the Seniors Independence Research Program-funded project exploring the support needs of elderly caregivers, a McMaster/University of Toronto study on the financial implications of early retirement for caregivers and the Canadian Study of Heath and Aging through Health Canada, in addition to countless requests from students in the fields of aging, wellness, women's studies, medicine, community health, and social work.

The Family Caregivers' Support Network has also been actively involved with the Metro Consumers of Long-Term Care, a group of over 200 senior individuals and groups educating other seniors on the implications of Long-Term Care reform. Working together to provide seniors with community information, educational workshops, and public forums, the collaboration has linked the Family Caregivers' Support Network with many senior caregivers and groups, strengthening caregiver participation in policy formation which directly affects their everyday caregiving.

In addition, the Family Caregivers' Support Network has been asked to join with the Mood Disorders Association of Toronto in providing workshops, resource packages, and support for family caregivers in the mental health community. These collaborative activities would be designed for senior caregivers of individuals suffering from depression and manic depression and caregivers suffering from depression themselves, two populations often marginalized and underserviced.

Since the inception of the project, staff and volunteers have also continued to meet with self-help and professionally led groups for caregivers as forums for talking with individual family caregivers from a variety of different backgrounds and with a variety of different support needs. It is these visits and ongoing consultation with individual family caregivers that provide the direction and focus for up-and-coming project activities, grounding the project activities in the needs of the community it supports.

DEVELOPMENT OF A SELF-HELP/ MUTUAL AID GROUP FOR PROFESSIONALS

Self-help groups for professionals were not considered in the original proposal to Health Canada, but have become one of the most important and successful activities of the Family Caregivers' Support Network. The twenty to thirty professionals who come to the monthly self-help "breakfast meetings" list their reasons for membership in the group as: "to share information and resources, to explore creative strategies to group work, to learn more about the role of mutual aid and support in our work with seniors, and to network and to support each other." One participant commented; "Our own support network will improve our work with caregivers and provide us with access to the insights, expertise and experiences of other workers in the field."

Breakfast meeting topics to date have included program evaluation, transitioning from professionally led groups to peer led, peer support resources, creative approaches to workshops for caregivers, language and cultural challenges in working with caregivers, as well as funding challenges.

Part peer support, part education, part networking, and part workshop, this new initiative falls into many activity areas. The meetings also follow a self-help model with shared leadership, information sharing, egalitarianism, peer support, and education. Confidentiality, documentation, and leadership are decided collectively, as is format and scheduling. Thus, as self-help activities assist family caregivers to support themselves and their loved ones, so they enable professional caregivers to do the same for their patients and clients, improving professional "care" and awareness of caregiving issues in the process.

DISCUSSION

Almost ten years ago, a group of frustrated caregivers designed a program which was driven by and designed to meet their needs. Part education, part mutual support, and part advocacy initiative, the program was unique in its mandate and broad in its proposed activities. After six years of funding negotiations, the network was born in the spring of 1995.

In one short year, the network staff, volunteers, and advisory committee members have managed to produce some startling results. Caregivers have developed their own support line, developed their own organizational structure, published their own newsletter, consulted on research and program planning while educating themselves on issues they choose to study and improving the understanding of professionals through the use of mutual-aid strategies.

The process of funding the network was not simple, as was illustrated by the "Storytelling" method. Implementation has also presented us with a number of challenges. Outreach to the isolated family caregiver has proven to be one of the greatest hurdles, but collaborations with home care and other home visiting associations have begun to access caregivers who may have no other contact with external support systems. In addition, growing media interest and coverage, including regular appearances on television and features in local and Ontariowide newspapers, have proven to be the most effective and cost-free method of promoting the workshops, the support line, and other supports offered by the network.

Other challenges include outreach to more ethnically diverse caregivers in ways which are compatible with their communities as well as continued advocacy efforts at a time when advocacy has never been more difficult nor more important in Ontario.

In addition to outreach challenges, we have not yet found a method that will ultimately and effectively capture all the outcomes, stories, successes, and challenges that implementation of this network has shown us, and we still have no clear idea of what the future of the network will look like. With seniors' health promotion programs being "sunsetted" across Canada, ongoing public funding for this program is insecure. The most pressing challenge of all then, is to enable caregivers to develop strong, sustainable, and visible network structure, able to take on the task of securing more public funds through ongoing campaigns and advocacy work or steering the network toward independent sources of income. As many of you already know, this route is always rocky, but given their record to date, the family caregivers involved in this new, unique, and very active work, are certainly ready for the challenge.

REFERENCES

Aronson, J. (1989). Family care of the elderly: Underlying assumptions and their consequences. *Canadian Journal on Aging, 4*(3): 115-125.

Aronson, J. (1992). Women's sense of responsibility for the care of old people: "But who else is going to do it?" *Gender and Society, 6*(1):8-29.

Barer, B.M. and Johnson, C. (1990). A critique of the caregiving literature. *The Gerontologist, 30*(1): 26-29.

Biegel, D.E., Shore, B.K., and Gordon, E. (Eds.) (1984). Family caregiver enhancement. *Building Support Networks for the Elderly: Theory and Applications.* London: Sage, 106-112.

Bornstein, J. (1994). Editorial: The caregiving dilemma. *The Canadian Journal on Aging, 13*(2): 129-141.

The Canadian Study of Health and Aging (1994). Patterns of caring for people with dementia in Canada. *Canadian Journal on Aging, 13*(4): 470-487.

Cohen, C.A., Gold, D.P., Shulman, K.I., and Zucchero, C.A. (1994). Positive aspects in caregiving: An overlooked variable in research. *Canadian Journal on Aging, 13*(3): 378-391.

Colantonio, A., Cohen, C., and Corlett, S. (1996). Self-help, mutual aid, and self-care: Self-help and mutual aid for elderly caregivers. *Symposium on Bridging Policy and Research on Aging in Canada.*

Feather, J. and Labonte, R. (1995). *Sharing Knowledge Gained from Health Promotion Practice.* Saskatoon, SK: Prairie Region Health Promotion Research Centre, University of Saskatchewan.

Fradkin, L. and Liberti, M. (1994). Caregiving. In P.B. Doress and D. Laskin Siegal (Eds.), *Ourselves, Growing Older.* Toronto: Touchstone, 214-218.

Guberman, N., Maheu, P., and Maille, C. (1992). Women as family caregivers: Why do they care? *The Gerontologist, 32*(5): 607-617.

Hartman, A. (1990). Aging as a family issue. *Social Work, 35*(5): 387-388.

Lavoie, J.P. (1995). Support groups for informal caregivers don't work! Refocus the groups or the evaluations? *Canadian Journal on Aging, 14*(3): 580-595.

Pearlin, L.I. (1992). Symposium: The careers of caregivers. *The Gerontologist, 32*(5): 647.

Rosenthal, C.J. and Gladstone, J. (1994). Family relationships and support in later life. In Victor W. Marshall and Barry D. McPherson (Eds.), *Aging: Canadian Perspectives*. Peterborough, Ontario: Broadview Press/Journal of Canadian Studies: 130-144.

Sokolovsky, J. (1990). Bringing culture back home: Aging, ethnicity and family support. In J. Sokolovsky (Ed.), *The Cultural Context of Aging*. New York: Bergen and Garvey, 68-72.

Stoller, E. (1990). Males as helpers: The role of sons, relatives and friends. *The Gerontologist, 30*(2): 228-234.

Whitlatch, Carol J., Zarit, S.H., and Von Eye, A. (1991). Efficacy of interventions with caregivers: A reanalysis. *The Gerontologist, 31*(1): 9-14.

Chapter 5

Some Important Areas of Group Work Expertise

John H. Ramey

As group workers, we have a tremendous opportunity and re-sponsibility to contribute to the quality of life for the people of our societies. We need to work together to expand recognition and understanding of our perception of how people can and should relate comfortably and productively together in corporate life, that is, group life outside the family.

We clearly recognize that participation in a group is "the heart of being social" and that work with groups really is the heart of doing social work. When AASWG first began to develop, it seemed to many of us to be a contradiction in terms that most of social work was being conceived as one-to-one (or at best, one-to-family) client-worker interaction. To most of us it was clear that social work has lost the soul of its purpose of building a brighter future for all people in our societies by helping them to work together in groups.

Broad social policy is as necessary at local, state, national, and international levels as are good public social support systems and one-to-one interpersonal interactions. But one of the two places where the real personal meaning and enjoyment of life is realized and the public considerations of problems and decisions are made is in the face-to-face group. (The other is, of course, the family.)

We know that there are certain values, knowledge, and skills which group workers bring to social work and to society. We also know that those perspectives which had been developed in the decades before NASW was formed were in danger of being aban-doned. Perhaps this abandonment was on purpose, perhaps not, but it was clear that we had to come together to rejuvenate group work and take it forward.

Thus we have spent most of the past two decades working together to create a new organization dedicated to the preservation and further development of group work practice within social work. This is not a recreation of the past. Too much has transpired in society, in social work, and in group work practice over the last forty some years. Yet, there is much more to be done. I appreciate this opportunity to reflect on our work and to make some suggestions for the future.

I will briefly touch on several areas of special expertise for group work: (1) democracy, (2) leadership development, (3) intergroup relations, (4) reduction of violence through conflict management, (5) play, (6) social action, (7) the enjoyment of life, (8) the importance of the group in a general developmental approach, and (9) understanding the group as a group. Some, if not most, of these areas are particular to group work and are not fully shared with the rest of social work. Emphasis on these areas is not intended to reduce the importance of the many other areas of modern group work development, only to emphasize some of those least recognized.

GROUP WORKERS KNOW
ABOUT DEMOCRATIC PROCESSES

In these days when democracy seems to be threatened around the world it is important to remind ourselves that as group workers we have commitment, expertise, and a long tradition as specialists in democratic processes.[1] This is inherent in the very idea that people come together in groups to work on their common concerns and those of the larger society. We really need to develop and emphasize this aspect of our work to our larger societies. We hear much about empowerment as a goal of social work but we know that this involves helping people learn how to function effectively in the groups which relate together as the decision-making units of our society. We know about roles, particularly leadership, group participation skills, responsibility, development of group activity content (action and other program agendas), use and resolution of conflict, and social action.

A particularly visible experience of group workers in action on behalf of democracy occurred right after World War II when Louis Lowy, Ruby Pernell, Margaret Berry, Ann Stencel, and many others worked with the U.S. High Commission in Germany and the State Department in replacing authoritarian style leadership with democratic style in work with youth groups. Group workers are carrying out similar projects even today.

We have also had a significant literature which dealt with the theme of group work's responsibilities in democracies. Some of these go back a few years but they include classics such as Grace Coyle's *Group Work and Democratic Values.*[2] And there are many other titles throughout the years that readily come to mind.

The development of democracy in groups is integral to the theme of the Ann Arbor Symposium: "Rebuilding Communities: The Challenges for Group Work."

GROUP WORKERS KNOW
ABOUT GROUP LEADERSHIP

Group workers know about another very important and related area of societal processes—group leadership.[3] There is a certain logic to following a discussion of democracy with one about competent leadership at the heart of democracy.

We know a lot about the development of group leaders. It is one role, among many, which members take in any activity of a functional group. Someone needs to take responsibility for helping a group organize, focus, and carry out the activities leading to the goals it has chosen after its leadership has helped it establish those goals. In current social work literature, too often the only reference is to the social-worker-as-leader even in relation to work with small groups. The worker's leadership skills, role modeling, etc., are discussed. These are very important, but it is even more significant when the worker does not have to be the group leader. It takes a lot of ego strength for a worker to assume such a modest behind-the-scenes role.

We know that in any group structure is required and that one key aspect of this structure is leadership. We know how to analyze the structure and help groups change structure to improve their accomplishments. Leadership can and probably should be situational. We have the opportunity to help various members take turns with leadership and other roles for various aspects of group life. Very few all-purpose leaders exist. It is relevant to the "empowerment" thrust in group work and social work today, but we do not often find client leadership role development as a central theme. Yet one of the needed outcomes of group work in central cities and minority communities is the development of knowledgeable, sensitive, caring, and competent leaders for the entire community from among the participants in our groups.

The responsibility for development of leadership among the members of the group we work with is another area most relevant to the theme of the Ann Arbor Symposium.

From a sociological view there is no physical social reality to "community." It is a concept. If there ever were a face-to-face community, today it is mostly a construct. We do not have town meetings anymore where all the residents of a community come together to discuss and take action on those issues which affect them. Thus, "community" is made up of many smaller face-to-face social units, groups, and families, whose leaders and members interact in a pattern of relationship which allows decisions to be made by representatives on behalf of the larger community interest. That is how our democracy works. But it requires leadership. When we do not develop leaders among our clients, their unique perspectives on the needs of society are not recognized in decision making.

Most important is the art of developing group leadership among the participants in the various groups with which we work. We need to pass the skill along. That is where we have lost our leadership in society. It is part of the loss which has led to political leadership with no experience, knowledge, or feeling for the problems faced by the minorities, immigrants, handicapped, women, homosexuals, and other outclasses of our society.

As group workers we have our challenges cut out for us. We need to focus on our own community leadership skills and involvement and on our skills in developing our clients' group leadership skills. We need to hurry along. Leadership on social issues is moving away from us all too quickly.

GROUP WORKERS KNOW
ABOUT INTERGROUP RELATIONS

If there is one area of need in our society today to which group work can bring its special knowledge and skill, it is that of intergroup relations.[4] Division and conflict among persons with distinct and claimed identities are rising throughout the world. Sometimes, as in the United States, it is described as differences in race. In other areas it is caste, nationality, religion, class, or family identity which brings hatred and keeps people apart.

Group work has a long history of working at helping people respect their heritages and identities and, at the same time, working on common interests with others in their neighborhoods, cities, and nations. One major value of group work has been the emphasis on inclusiveness. Knowledge and skill in the processes of forming groups and working with them toward greater understanding and achievement are one core aspect of group work. We understand and can work with intrapsychic dynamics, cultural and community factors, and group processes. We have a long-respected tradition of knowledge, skill, and experience in this area which needs to be extended and enhanced in coming years.

Intergroup relations so overrides other problems in most societies, and particularly here in the United States, that the impact of actions in professional practice must always be measured against the potential for positive or negative impact. Very little, if any, neutral ground is found here, and one must choose the positive road.

The organizers of AASWG understood the imperative to deal professionally, personally, and organizationally with the issues of race, class, and nationality. In recent years AASWG's Committee on Diversity has worked to find ways of responding in practice, education, research, and professional areas to expand our commitment to diversity.

We have so much to offer in this needy area of society that we really must give it frontline attention. Too many forces are working to divide and separate us from one another. We are in "an international professional organization" for social purpose, practice, and education. Let's see what we can do in the future to make a real difference, an improvement.

GROUP WORKERS KNOW ABOUT THE REDUCTION OF VIOLENCE AND CONFLICT MANAGEMENT

All conflict is not bad. In fact, as we know, conflict is important for decision making and change, and for growth. On the other hand, undirected and uncontrolled conflict can be destructive to groups and communities. We are specialists in conflict management and resolution and should present ourselves to groups and communities as such when the need arises. In the areas of street gangs and civil rights, many of us worked to bring about constructive resolution to the violent and combative confrontations. These are played out continuously in schools, at work, in community agencies, and in politics.

GROUP WORKERS KNOW ABOUT PLAY

We know that play is rehearsal for real life. It models interaction, attitudes, decision-making processes, and conflict resolution in situations that are not life-outcome threatening. It helps develop skills. This is true whether the groups are composed of children, adults, teenagers, or senior citizens. Play has been rediscovered, but is now called "play therapy."

After the integrated methods approaches were adopted and group work curricula were subject to the approval of all faculty in the schools rather than group work faculty, the word was out that all courses that contained group activities were to be eliminated. Considered "play," not "work," they were dismissed from the curriculum. We need to reintroduce and develop support for the content knowledge and skills of "play" activity in groups for the modern era.

GROUP WORKERS KNOW ABOUT INVOLVING PEOPLE IN SOCIAL ACTION

As a matter of fact, it can be said that the ultimate outcome of all group process is to encourage and support people's collective abilities to take charge of their own lives. Much of this does not necessarily involve influencing the body politic, but much of it does.

When necessary, groups should be encouraged and prepared to express their experiences and viewpoints in public decision-making forums, and directly to the decision makers and administrators in constructive ways.

Much literature exists on working with social action groups. One memorable work is *Group Work and Social Action*, co-edited by Abe Vinik and the late Morris Levin.[5] We need to put forth our knowledge and responsibility in teaching and practice for social action groups.

GROUP WORKERS KNOW HOW TO HELP PEOPLE ENJOY LIFE

I remember a caseworker challenging group workers by suggesting that the people in the groups were "having fun" and, therefore, the work could not be serious and, above all, it could not be social work. Their approach was that all must be serious and somber. We know that people learn more from pleasurable experiences. We also recognize, as previously stated, that play prepares people, as individuals and in groups, to work together on the more serious issues of community life. We also believe that life should basically be enjoyable. Among other contexts we work in are the mental health institutions. Here society has gathered individuals and groups for whom there is often no joy in life.

Group activities reinforce the joy of life. In the various types of community centers we work to maintain, enhance, and share the cultural heritages of our members and neighbors. Most of these activities are basically enjoyable. Properly understood and worked with, however, they are powerful activities for achievement of many individual, group, and community goals.

GROUP WORKERS KNOW ABOUT THE IMPORTANCE OF THE GROUP IN A GENERAL DEVELOPMENTAL APPROACH

The original model of group work was developmental. We worked in settings that focused upon achieving behavior and attitudinal goals, rather than on defined, existing problems. This interaction was considered productive and enhanced the life chances of the group members in normal settings. This was the orientation even if the groups were what would be defined today as deviant or dysfunctional. The emphasis was on the positive. Our society's loss of focus on what should be positive life achievements for children, youth, adults, and seniors is partly the result of our shift to an exclusively problem-centered approach. We were moved from a developmental model to a residual model without understanding the implications of this move. In part it was a political process, too. We were merged with the much more conservatively oriented and politically dominant casework organizations who considered our social activism threatening. Theirs was a residual approach.

It is interesting that we shifted from an emphasis on healthy development to solving problems and that now society is shifting back to emphasis on creating well-being. The recognition is that one cannot always remedy situations which were allowed to become problems. We should shift at least a major part of our efforts back to the developmental approach.

One of the major thrusts of the recent study funded by the Carnegie Corporation of youth at risk is that we need to devote more of our resources to helping youth grow up in normal, constructive lifestyles.[6] The Youth Leadership Training Project of the Northeast Ohio chapter addresses this need directly by providing training for the workers with youth groups in all kinds of settings. It is very encouraging to note that among our members a number work in camps, community centers, schools, and other settings where the general thrust is developmental. It is important that the staff be social workers, however, because always in these settings individuals and groups need special help in functioning and a general social goals model is needed for such settings, not just recreation for recreation's sake.

GROUP WORKERS KNOW HOW
TO UNDERSTAND THE GROUP AS A GROUP

One fact that is least understood by nongroup workers trying to work with groups, is that the group is an entity in and of itself, made up of, but separate from, the individuals who are its members. If it is a group and the worker is successful, the group owns the group.

This can be an area of real challenge, requiring some modification of outlook in secure treatment or involuntary settings such as juvenile detention centers. In such settings all outcomes a group might seek to achieve will not be possible.

In this brief presentation, I cannot fully develop any one of these themes but merely suggest that they are important areas for development of group work teaching, practice, research, and publication.

Several areas of AASWG's structure and role in group work need special attention and development: (1) research and teaching, (2) ethics, (3) chapter development, and (4) the international scope of AASWG. Special recognition needs to be given to the type of organizational structure that is appropriate to group work and AASWG and to the international character of AASWG in this shrinking world—the use of modern technology to maintain connections and accomplish the work of the organization. These will have to wait for a future discussion.

In his book *Social Welfare: From Charity to Justice*, John M. Romanyshyn says, "All around us there are signs that human beings are coming alive to new and exciting potentialities in the nature of man and the possibilities for social life. Man was made for joy, for creation of meaning, for ritual and drama, for love, for poetry and mystery, for self-transcendence, and for union with all mankind. There is more, much more, to man than the narrow image of him that we have incorporated into our economic and political life. Here lies the hope for human welfare."[7]

We believe that effective group work holds the key to the development that Romanyshyn so eloquently projects for the future of mankind in all societies. That is the challenge of group workers in rebuilding communities.

NOTES

1. Adapted from *Social Work with Groups Newsletter*, April 1996, pp. 1, 13.
2. Coyle, Grace. (1947). *Group Work and Democratic Values*. New York: The Woman's Press.
3. Adapted from *Social Work with Groups Newsletter*, July 1996, pp. 1-3.
4. Adapted from *Social Work with Groups Newsletter*, December 1995/January 1996, pp. 10-22.

5. Vinik, Abe and Morris Levin (Eds.) (1991). *Social Action in Group Work.* Binghamton, NY: The Haworth Press, Inc. (Also published as *Social Work with Groups*, Vol. 14, Nos. 3/4, 1991.)

6. Carnegie Corporation of New York. (1992) *A Matter of Time: Risk and Opportunity in the Nonschool Hours.* New York: Carnegie Corporation of New York.

7. Romanyshyn, John M., with the assistance of Annie L. Romanyshyn. (1971). *Social Welfare: From Charity to Justice.* New York: Random House, p. 408.

SECTION III:
PAPERS

Chapter 6

AIDS Prevention for Adults with Serious Mental Illness: Improving Perceived Sexual Self-Efficacy

Meredith Hanson

Adults with serious and persistent mental illness are highly vulnerable to HIV infection (Carey et al., 1997; McKinnon et al., 1996). Due to sequelae of mental disorders such as impulsiveness and impaired judgment, many clients of mental health facilities are apt to engage in HIV/AIDS risk-related activities (Carmen and Brady, 1990). One study, for example, found that 19 percent of the patients on an acute care psychiatric ward engaged in HIV risk-related behaviors (Sacks, Silberstein, et al., 1990). Another investigation discovered that 42 percent of the adults admitted to an acute care psychiatric facility reported HIV risk-related behaviors during the five years preceding their hospitalization (Sacks, Perry, et al., 1990).

Reports from psychiatric hospitals reveal HIV-seropositive rates of between 5 percent and 14 percent among psychiatric inpatients (Cournos et al., 1991; Volavka et al., 1991;1992). Surveys of mental health clinics find that clients are misinformed about HIV/AIDS and engage in activities such as substance use, unprotected sex, receptive anal sex, and sex with injection drug users, that place them at high-risk for HIV infection (Goisman et al., 1991; Hanson et al., 1992; Kalichman et al., 1994; Kelly et al., 1995; Steiner, Lussier, and Rosenblatt, 1992). Adults with serious mental disorders also seem more concerned than other community members about the risks for HIV infection, and they are comparatively less self-confident that they can avoid infection (Cates, Bond, and Graham, 1994).

Clearly, members of this client population would benefit from AIDS education and prevention. Despite their need, few evaluations of potentially useful strategies have been published (Cournos and Bakalar, 1996). Carmen and Brady (1990) described a drop-in group that was well received by members of an inner-city mental health clinic. Meyer and colleagues (1992) reported that individuals who were hospitalized on an acute psychiatric admission ward improved their knowledge and decreased nonfunctional attitudes about HIV/AIDS following a seven-week HIV prevention group. Hanson and co-workers (1994) and Rolon, Cancel, and Hanson (1993) found that outpatients with coexisting substance use and mental disorders (dual diagnoses) who completed a nine-session AIDS prevention group acquired knowledge about condom use, used condoms more often, reduced risky sexual practices, and became more assertive in sexual encounters. Cates and Graham (1993) reported, however, that a three-session HIV/AIDS education program delivered to residents of community mental health group homes did not produce significant changes in knowledge or attitudes about HIV/AIDS. In none of the interventions was AIDS education associated with such untoward side effects as sexual acting out, psychiatric decompensation, or increases in HIV risk-related behaviors.

This chapter reports on a nine-session AIDS prevention group (Hanson, Cancel, and Rolon, 1994). Unlike previous interventions, this group focused on facilitating changes in perceived sexual self-efficacy, as well as actual behavior. Self-efficacy is a construct that is grounded in social learning and cognitive behavioral theory. It is the belief that one can and should be in control in particular situations. Essentially a performance expectation, it can be thought of as people's confidence in their ability to organize and enact courses of action that are needed to attain particular performances (Bandura, 1986; 1990). Self-efficacy affects behavior by mediating effort and persistence (Annis and Davis, 1988; Jemmott et al., 1992).

Improving perceived sexual self-efficacy is a necessary element in AIDS risk reduction (Catania, Kegeles, and Coates, 1990). Persons who do not feel self-efficacious are unlikely to adopt protective behaviors even if they know that those behaviors will reduce their risk of HIV infection. For example, clients may know that using latex condoms will reduce HIV transmission. They will not use condoms, however, it they do not perceive that they are capable of persuading their sexual partners to use them. In addition, they probably will continue unprotected sexual activities if they do not believe that they have the capacity to refuse unprotected sex.

CONCEPTUAL FRAMEWORK

The AIDS prevention group was grounded in several complementary theories, including social learning theory, health psychology, the health belief model, and empowerment theory (Bandura, 1986; Becker and Joseph, 1988; Catania, Kegeles, and Coates, 1990; Lee, 1994; Manning, 1998). It employed prevention strategies found to be useful with other populations who engage in behaviors that place them at risk for HIV infection (Kelly, 1995; Schilling et al., 1991).

Consistent with this conceptual framework, it was postulated that individuals must go through several stages to alter behaviors and attitudes that place them at risk for HIV infection. First, they must understand how AIDS is transmitted, perceive that the risk is serious, and believe that they are vulnerable. Second, they must learn about effective risk strategies, have confidence that those strategies can reduce the risk of infection, and believe that they can implement those strategies. Third, they must have an opportunity to learn and practice those strategies. Fourth, they must receive positive feedback, mutual aid, and support from their peers, which reinforce the use of the protective strategies (Bandura, 1990; Catania, Kegeles, and Coates, 1990; Gibson, Catania, and Peterson, 1991; Gilchrist and Schinke, 1983; Kelly et al., 1995).

METHOD

Sample

Clients of a hospital-based, inner-city day program for adults with dual diagnoses were surveyed to ascertain their knowledge of HIV/AIDS and the nature of their risk-related behaviors (Hanson et al., 1992). Following this needs assessment, which revealed that they were at risk for HIV infection primarily through heterosexual activities (e.g., unprotected sex, multiple sex partners), individuals were recruited for a nine-session AIDS prevention group. Clients were informed that participation was voluntary and that the group's purpose was to teach them more about HIV/AIDS, including how to protect their partners and themselves from infection during sexual encounters.

Thirty-one people were interested in the group. Eleven were selected systematically for the group's first cycle. Candidates' names were alphabetized in separate lists for men and women. Every third person was selected from each list until eleven people were enrolled. (One group member, who graduated from the day program before her post-group interview, is not included in this report.) Group size was established to conform with the sizes of other groups in the day program. Clients who were not admitted to the group's first cycle were enrolled in subsequent cycles of the group. Group members were comparable to other clients of the day program in their demographic characteristics, psychiatric diagnoses, and substance use patterns with one exception. To ensure an adequate number of women in the group, they were overrepresented in the group's composition, compared to their numbers in the day program. (A mixed-gender group was formed to address stereotypical beliefs that the men and women had about each other and to facilitate the development of heterosexual communication skills.)

Seven men and three women entered the group. Their mean age was 37.7 years (range: 31-52). They had completed an average of 11.5 grades in school. Seven were African American; two were Latino; one was white. One was married and living with her spouse. All were sexually active. All received public assistance or Supplementary Security Income. All members, except one alcohol-dependent woman, had histories of polysubstance abuse. All had past psychiatric hospitalizations. Six were diagnosed with schizophrenic disorders; two had bipolar disorders; one was diagnosed with major depression; and one was diagnosed with schizoaffective disorder. Group members were psychiatrically stable and abstinent from alcohol and illicit drugs when the group began.

Procedure

Prior to starting the group, and within two weeks of its completion, all members were interviewed and completed a 20-item, Likert-like sexual self-efficacy scale (El-Bassel and Schilling, 1993). The scale included statements about discussing safer sex with sexual partners and implementing protective strategies (e.g., wearing condoms.) In individual interviews the clients were asked to think about each of the twenty statements and decide whether they could do what was described. They were assured that there were no right or wrong answers. Reliability analysis revealed that the sexual self-efficacy scale had high internal consistency: baseline, coefficient alpha $=$ .88; post-group $-$.81. Thus, summative scale scores were used in the analysis.

The Preventive Intervention

The group was co-led by a female AIDS educator and a male social worker. It met one hour per week for nine weeks. Through didactic presentations, role-plays with videotaped feedback, and group discussion, participants were taught protective strategies they could use in sexual encounters, and they practiced problem solving and decision making. Clients learned how to recognize specific situations in which they placed themselves at risk for HIV infection, avoid those situations in the future, develop refusal skills and other ways to handle pressures to resume risky sexual activities, and identify social supports for maintaining safer sexual practices (Rolon, Cancel, and Hanson, 1993).

The first two group sessions introduced the group's purpose and encouraged participants to discover how they were vulnerable for HIV infection by helping them identify specific sexual situations in which they were at risk for infection. In sessions three through five, using situations they generated, members learned and practiced assertiveness and decision-making strategies such as refusing unprotected sexual activity, initiating discussions of safer sexual practices, and suggesting alternatives to unprotected sex. Role-plays were videotaped to give members a chance to observe their actions and to receive feedback from others. Sessions six and seven focused on using condoms and latex dams (for oral sex). Group members learned how to put on latex condoms, use water-based lubricants, and construct latex dams from condoms. The last two sessions linked risky sexual practices to substance use and underscored the need for mutual support and ongoing vigilance to sustain safer sexual practices. In all of the sessions participants received positive feedback and encouragement aimed at reinforcing their beliefs that they could enact the different protective strategies competently.

RESULTS

The Wilcoxon Matched-Pairs Signed-Ranks test showed that the group members' total perceived self-efficacy scores increased significantly by the group's end ($Z = - 2.67$, $p<.01$). The self-efficacy scores for nine members increased by an average of 25 percent. The tenth member's score remained unchanged.

Changes in perceived sexual self-efficacy were more remarkable for the three women in the group than for the men. At the group's start women felt slightly less sexually self-confident than did men. By the group's end they reported feeling more confidant in sexual situations than did the men. (Due to the small numbers involved statistical analyses were not conducted.)

At the group's start the members felt least confident in areas including resisting unprotected and unwanted sex once encounters started and using condoms during oral and vaginal sex. They were more confident in their abilities to avoid unprotected sex before encounters started. By the group's finish they gained confidence in their abilities to stop sexual encounters that were leading to unsafe sex. They still expressed doubts about their abilities to initiate discussions of safer sexual practices and to use condoms during oral sex, however.

The clients' self-reports suggested that their behavior changed as their confidence grew. Several months after the group's conclusion they continued to report that they were avoiding risky sexual situations. They also were more likely to request condoms from the day program's nurse than they were before they entered the group. Staff members, as well as clients, reported no untoward incidents or psychiatric decompensation related to group involvement.

DISCUSSION AND IMPLICATIONS
FOR SOCIAL WORK PRACTICE WITH GROUPS

Competence in high-risk sexual situations is a function of personal capacities, environmental resources, and motivation (Maluccio and Libassi, 1984). Generally, people strengthen their competence and gain mastery in their lives in social contexts, in which norms and beliefs are altered, new skills are learned, and new behaviors are reinforced. The results of this study show that through their involvement in AIDS prevention groups, adults with serious mental illness can develop confidence in their abilities to handle sexual encounters and resist pressures to engage in unprotected sex; they can learn new protective strategies; and they can develop a support system that helps them maintain behavioral and attitudinal changes.

Several suggestions for social work practice with groups emerge from this study. First, it is crucial that group leaders help members identify the specific sexual situations that place them at risk for HIV infection and help them learn new skills relevant to those situations. Groups provide excellent contexts for observational learning (Toseland and Rivas, 1998). For participants to become motivated to adopt new skills, however, they must believe that the skills apply to the sexual situations they face. They also must see that other group members have acquired the skills and that they have used them successfully (Bandura, 1986). Thus, group leaders must give members chances to see others use new skills and be reinforced for using them. Videotaping is an excellent tool for allowing members to see the results of their efforts immediately and for enabling them to receive feedback from their peers. The interaction that occurs around the videotaping provides numerous opportunities for informal feedback and for helping members to learn new skills by observing the actions of others. These opportunities to practice and receive feedback about protective strategies are the most direct ways to influence members' self-confidence (perceived self-efficacy) and to support behavioral change (Bandura, 1990; Gilchrist et al., 1986).

Second, group participation validates the members' experiences that sexual encounters are stressful. As the group develops, members begin to discuss their fears about practicing safer sex. In particular, they express worries about rejection and about other forms of retaliation (e.g., physical abuse). When these concerns are raised it is important for the group leaders to encourage the members to discuss them and to help them problem solve to handle them. Through these discussions the members' sense of social isolation decreases, and they receive encouragement for asserting themselves. This support was especially apparent among the women group members. Several of them commented that the group was the only place where they were listened to by people who know what they are going through. Both men and women developed a sense of mutuality and support in the group that extended outside the group and helped them to persist when faced with extreme anxiety and concern.

A final suggestion concerns the time-limited nature of the group. Because the group is short term, it is necessary for the group leaders to be active and structured in their approach. Discussion of client concerns has to be balanced with the need to cover group content in a timely manner. This dilemma was addressed in the AIDS prevention group by encouraging the group members to meet outside formal group meeting times and to bring questions back to the group. Since the group took place in a day program, group members had many chances to meet with each other outside the group. These extra-group meetings enabled the members to strengthen their mutual support. They also provided them with a means for continuing to meet informally after the group ended, which probably contributed to the group's ongoing beneficial impact.

The findings of this study are exploratory in nature. They are limited by a small sample size and no control group. They suggest, however, promising avenues for future practice and research to help persons with serious mental illness reduce their risks for HIV infection.

REFERENCES

Annis, H.M. and Davis, C.S. (1988). Assessment of expectancies. In D.M. Donovan and G.A. Marlatt (Eds.), *Assessment of Addictive Behaviors* (pp. 84-111). New York: Guilford.

Bandura, A. (1986). *Social Foundations of Thought and Action: A Social Cognitive Theory.* Englewood Cliffs, NJ: Prentice-Hall.

Bandura, A. (1990). Perceived self-efficacy in the exercise of control over AIDS infection. *Evaluation and Program Planning, 13*(1), 1-17.

Becker, M.H. and Joseph, J.G. (1988). AIDS and behavioral change to reduce risk: A review. *American Journal of Public Health, 78*(3), 394-410.

Carey, M.P., Carey, K.B., Weinhardt, L.S., and Gordon, C.M. (1997). Behavioral risk for HIV infection among adults with a severe and persistent mental illness: Patterns and psychological antecedents. *Community Mental Health Journal, 33*(2), 133-142.

Carmen, E. and Brady, S.M. (1990). AIDS risk and prevention for the chronic mentally ill. *Hospital and Community Psychiatry, 41*(6), 652-657.

Catania, J.A., Kegeles, S.M., and Coates, T.J. (1990). Towards an understanding of risk behavior: An AIDS risk reduction model (ARRM). *Health Education Quarterly, 17*(1), 53-72.

Cates, J.A., Bond, G.R., and Graham, L.L. (1994). AIDS knowledge, attitudes, and risk behavior among people with serious mental illness. *Psychosocial Rehabilitation Journal, 17*(4), 19-29.

Cates, J.A. and Graham, L.L. (1993). HIV and serious mental illness: Reducing the risk. *Community Mental Health Journal, 29*(1), 35-47.

Cournos, F. and Bakalar, N. (Eds.) (1996). *AIDS and People with Severe Mental Illness: A Handbook for Mental Health Professionals.* New Haven, CT: Yale University Press.

Cournos, F., Empfield, M., Horwath, E., McKinnon, K., Meyer, I., Schrage, H., Currie, C., and Agosin, B. (1991). HIV seroprevalence among patients admitted to two psychiatric hospitals. *American Journal of Psychiatry, 148*(9), 1225-1230.

El-Bassel, N. and Schilling, R.S. (1993). Sexual self-efficacy questionnaire. Columbia University School of Social Work.

Gibson, D.R., Catania, J.A., and Peterson, J.L. (1991). Theoretical background. In J.L. Sorensen, L.A. Wermuth, D.R. Gibson, K-H. Choi, J.R. Guydish, and S.L. Batki (Eds.), *Preventing AIDS in Drug Users and Their Sexual Partners* (pp. 62-74). New York: Guilford.

Gilchrist, L.D. and Schinke, S.P. (1983). Coping with contraception: Cognitive and behavioral methods with adolescents. *Cognitive Therapy and Research, 7*(5), 379-388.

Gilchrist, L.D., Schinke, S.P., Bobo, J.K., and Snow, W.H. (1986). Self-control skills for preventing smoking. *Addictive Behaviors. 11*(2), 169-174.

Goisman, R.M., Kent, A.B., Montgomery, E.C., and Cheevers, M.M. (1991). AIDS education for patients with chronic mental illness. *Community Mental Health Journal, 27*(3), 189-197.

Hanson, M., Cancel, J., and Rolon, A. (1994). Reducing AIDS risks among dually disordered adults. *Research on Social Work Practice, 4*(1), 14-27.

Hanson, M., Kramer, T.H., Gross, W., Qunitana, J., Li, P-W, and Asher, R. (1992). AIDS awareness and risk behaviors among dually disordered adults. *AIDS Education and Prevention, 4*(1), 41-51.

Jemmott, J.B. III, Jemmott, L.W., Spears, H., Hewitt, N., and Cruz-Collins, M. (1992). Self-efficacy, hedonistic expectancies, and condom-use intentions among inner-city black adolescent women: A social cognitive approach to AIDS risk behavior. *Journal of Adolescent Health, 13*(6), 512-519.

Kalichman, S.C., Kelly, J.A., Johnson, J.R., and Bulto, M. (1994). Factors associated with risk for HIV infection among chronic mentally ill adults. *American Journal of Psychiatry, 151*(2), 221-227.

Kelly, J.A. (1995). *Changing HIV Risk Behavior: Practical Strategies*. New York: Guilford.

Kelly, J.A., Murphy, D.A., Sikkema, K.J., Somlai, A.M., Mulry, G.W., Fernandez, M.I., Miller, J.G., and Stevenson, L.Y. (1995). Predictors of high and low levels of HIV risk behavior among adults with chronic mental illness. *Psychiatric Services, 46*(8), 813-818.

Lee, J.A.B. (1994). *The Empowerment Approach to Social Work Practice*. New York: Columbia University Press.

Maluccio, A.N. and Libassi, M.F. (1984). Competence clarification in social work practice. *Social Thought, 10*(2), 51-58.

Manning, S.S. (1998). Empowerment in mental health programs: Listening to the voices. In L.M. Gutierrez, R.J. Parsons, and E.O. Cox (Eds.), *Empowerment in Social Work Practice: A Sourcebook* (pp. 89-109). Pacific Grove, CA: Brooks/ Cole.

McKinnon, K., Cournos, F., Sugden, R., Guido, J.R., and Herman, R. (1996). The relative contributions of psychiatric symptoms and AIDS knowledge to HIV risk behaviors among people with severe mental illness. *Journal of Clinical Psychiatry, 57*(11), 506-513.

Meyer, I., Cournos, F., Empfield, M., Agosin, B., and Floyd, P. (1992). HIV prevention among psychiatric inpatients: A pilot risk-reduction study. *Psychiatric Quarterly, 63*(2), 187-197.

Rolon, A., Cancel, J., and Hanson, M. (1993). An AIDS awareness and prevention group for dually disordered adults. *TIE Lines, 10*(3), 6-8.

Sacks, M.H., Perry, S., Graver, R., Shindeldecker, R., and Hall, S. (1990). Self-reported HIV-related risk behaviors in acute psychiatric inpatients: A pilot study. *Hospital and Community Psychiatry, 41*(11), 1253-1255.

Sacks, M., Silberstein, C., Weiler, P., and Perry, S. (1990). HIV-related risk factors in acute psychiatric inpatients. *Hospital and Community Psychiatry, 41*(4), 449-451.

Schilling, R.S., El-Bassel, N., Schinke, S.P., Gordon, K., and Nichols, S. (1991). Building skills of recovering women drug users to reduce heterosexual AIDS transmission: *Public Health Reports, 106*(2), 297-304.

Steiner, J., Lussier, R., and Rosenblatt, W. (1992). Knowledge about and risk factors for AIDS in a day hospital population. *Hospital and Community Psychiatry, 43*(7), 734-735.

Toseland, R.W. and Rivas, R.F. (1998). *An Introduction to Group Work Practice*. Third Edition. Boston: Allyn and Bacon.

Volavka, J., Convit, A., Czobor, P., Douyon, R., O'Donnell, J., and Ventura, F. (1991). HIV seroprevalence and risk behaviors in psychiatric inpatients. *Psychiatry Research, 39*(2), 109-114.

Volavka, J. Convit, A., O'Donnell, J., Douyon, R., Evangelista, C., and Czobor, P. (1992). Assessment of risk behaviors for HIV infection among psychiatric inpatients. *Hospital and Community Psychiatry, 43*(5), 482-485.

Chapter 7

But Does It Really Work Like That? Verifying a Piece of Social Group Work Theory

Sue Henry
Satish K. Nair

We are at a time—and our theory building is at a stage—of conceptualization in social work with groups, to work more proactively at verifying pieces of theory. Recent advances in research methods, and systematic reports of practice experience at these symposia and in the group work journal make it possible to explore new ways of building our knowledge base.

We have more tools at our command than in previous times, to validate what we do and what we know. In this chapter, verification of one small, albeit important piece of group work practice theory will be demonstrated: the pregroup interview in which an initial working agreement is formed. The theory-building tool used in verifying this piece of social group work theory is the qualitative data analysis program, NUDIST (for *N*onnumerical *U*nstructured *D*ata *I*ndexing *S*earching and *T*heorizing), which will be discussed later.

The notion of a pregroup interview entered my (Henry) understanding of group work practice at the Alta Social Settlement House in Cleveland. Composition of each group at the house was designed following interviews of children and youth members of the settlement. The interviews were conducted by the house permanent staff. Goals that the house members wanted to work on or achieve in their "club" were elicited, and assignment to a specific group was made on the basis of age, developmental level, and homogeneity of "purposes." A rudimentary "group contract" ensued from this interview and was refined and polished in subsequent discussions between the members and the worker. That kernel of an idea about how to begin with a group seemed so good that I have incorporated it into my practice, writing, teaching, and research ever since. The idea itself has been refined and tested over time, and is now at the heart of this chapter.

What was (initially, in my practice) this rudimentary "group contract" has been expanded to a more formal contract, and has been the subject of research and writing (Henry, 1972; Estes and Henry, 1976; Henry, 1981; Henry, 1992). Now, the pregroup interview, and the negotiation of a reciprocal contract are linked, as an initial phase of practice. The pregroup interview is a process different from the intake interview by which a person comes into agency service. The pregroup interview is held with each prospective member of a group for the purpose of clarifying what the worker and the members each may expect from the other, the usual requirements to which each may be held, and other factors that bind them together (Schwartz, 1962, p. 174). It is recommended that the pregroup interview be conducted by the person who will be the worker with the group and not by any other staff member. In the case of co-workers, both may participate in the interviews, although not necessarily at the same time.

The literature of social group work has long shown the value of establishing a contract between members and of prospective members of a group and the worker; among the members, as the collective entity, "group," and between them collectively and the worker; and among all the members and the worker. The contract conforms to social group work's historic commitment to equalize, as far as possible, the power balance between member(s) and worker.

Garvin presented the contract as having:

. . . roots in social work's commitments to the self-determination of the client so that the client is not manipulated toward ends (s)he does not seek through means (s)he does not accept. (Garvin, 1969, p. 128)

Hartford reported the appearance of the use of a contract, albeit not labeling the practice as such, in her paper at the NASW Tenth Anniversary Symposium:

> There is increasing evidence that social group workers are making use of a concept of goals at a deliberate and conscious level. The worker and members verbalize what they wish to achieve in a group. From a treatment standpoint, this means bringing to awareness of all parties of the process, in and through the group experience, the direction toward which they are moving . . .
> . . . On the basis of this premise, it would then follow that every action by the worker, every piece of program introduced or encouraged, whether it is discussion or activity, the choice and use of facilities, meeting time, and even the group composition itself, would be a calculated and planned action based on some objective which is understood not only by the worker but also by group members and agreed upon by them. (Hartford, 1966, p. 138)

Social work and other theorists have noted the properties of an agreement that resembles what is here referred to as a group contract. Work by Garvin (1969), Hartford (1966, 1972), Cartwright and Zander (1960), Schopler and Galinsky (1974), Mills (1967), and Henry (1972, 1974, 1981, 1992) combine to explain what the ingredients of that agreement are—the contract terms. In the original work on which this chapter is based, nine contract terms were derived from the theoretical literature and from research. Those nine terms are:

1. the direction the group is moving (Hartford, 1966)
2. group as a unit as referent (Mills, 1967)
3. member behavior (Garvin, 1969)
4. program (discussion or activity) (Hartford, 1966, Cartwright and Zander, 1960)
5. worker behavior (Hartford, 1966; Garvin, 1969)
6. choice and use of facilities (Hartford, 1966)
7. meeting time and number of meetings (Hartford, 1966)
8. membership policies (open or closed in terms of membership
9. how members are added or dropped (Hartford, 1966)

In work previously developed, I portrayed the pregroup interview as consisting of a set of procedures, incorporating particular content, arriving at an initial working agreement through the use of specific skills (Henry, 1992, p. 52). The agreement (or contract) that is formulated during the interview is the outcome of the interview. I call this the Reciprocal Contract. This contract:

> . . . is agreed between each prospective group member and the group worker (Henry, 1992, p. 54) and states that what the person needs to work on can be appropriated into the generalized initial group purpose. The worker agrees (or not) with the prospective member that the group can serve her or his stated needs. (Estes and Henry, 1976; Garvin, 1969; Henry, 1992)

An example of such a negotiation conducted through a pregroup interview and the ensuing Reciprocal Contract may be seen in the following excerpt from a group practice record.

I met with Jane D. in a pregroup interview to assess suitability for the court-ordered domestic violence/parenting group. After a brief introduction and welcome process, I proceeded to discuss the purpose of the group with Jane D. I explained that the group was designed for women who had been arrested for domestic violence and who also needed a special focus on parenting issues. Jane was quiet at the beginning and appeared to be listening attentively to the information given.

Jane had a few questions about the number of women in the group and the cost involved, so we discussed these issues and I asked her if she had any more questions before we moved ahead. We continued with the interview and I asked Jane about herself and the incident that brought her into the court system. Jane was very verbal and expressive in her explanation of the incident. I went on to ask her more questions to help determine suitability.

I then discussed with Jane the procedures and methods used in group and how the groups are structured. I explained that we begin group with a check-in process of the week and move into a topic of discussion. I explained that participation is a very important part of the process and often times homework is given to help facilitate learning.

The next part of the interview involved the discussion of style and how Jane will get the most out of a group process. I explained my style of work to Jane, describing my nature as a worker and how I facilitate group meetings. I explained that I allow the group to flow as it will and that I do not try to fill every moment of the group with information and conversation; I allow for silences and internal processes of the group members. Jane shared that she had never been involved in a group before, but that she seemed to be comfortable around others. We discussed the issue of whether my style would work for her in this setting and came to the agreement that she would be appropriate for group. Because this is a court-ordered situation, Jane did not have a choice whether to join a group, but she did have a choice of which group she would like to join, and what agency.

Jane and I proceeded to go over the written contract for a new group member. In this, the group rules and guidelines are discussed, including issues such as financial commitments and confidentiality. I discussed with Jane the importance of the group being a safe place. Jane and I went over each area of the contract, making sure that each topic was covered and understood. The final part of the contract focused on her goals and objectives and we proceeded to fill out this section together. Jane said one her goals was to learn more about the way in which domestic violence affects her children.

I ended the interview by giving Jane the information necessary for her to attend the first group meeting. She appeared to be relaxed by the end of the interview and said that even though she is not happy about being ordered to attend thirty-six weeks of group, the experience will most likely benefit her and her children.

The records of the pregroup interviews referred to in this chapter were analyzed using a computer-based qualitative data analysis program called NUDIST. It is a computer package designed to aid in analyzing nonnumerical and unstructured data. Among other things, it is an electronic technology form of the Content Analysis technique. The process records which were used came from students in a Social Work with Groups class at the University of Denver's graduate School of Social Work. All conventions of confidentiality and agency permission were observed.

NUDIST can handle data such as transcripts of unstructured interviews, minutes of meetings, field notes, newspaper clippings, and historical documents, as well as process recordings of social work practice incidents. It enables a researcher to manage, explore, and search the text of documents, test theories about data, and generate reports, including statistical summaries. This is achieved using a process of document and indexing database creation. The document database provides a system to manage data documents by allowing storing and retrieval of documents on line, writing and editing memos regarding ideas that emerge from the documents, and searching for actual words or phrases in the text of the documents that are automatically indexed.

The indexing database provides the user with the means to categorize, code, and index documents. This database permits the user to create categories that reflect themes from the document, sort and re-sort data and indexes to locate patterns, index segments of text from the data under various categories, and report all references of actual text under each index from various documents.

The pregroup interviews used in this study were transcribed and converted into documents in the particular format that NUDIST recognizes. All of the interviews were then introduced into NUDIST as different documents of the same analysis project. The emphasis, in this analysis, was placed on the drawing of themes and concepts from the documents. This was done by using NUDIST and generating in vivo categories to group each of the statements/sentences/text units in the data. These categories were then analyzed for common characteristics and grouped together under an index that represented a higher order of abstraction. This process of indexing by abstraction was continued until all the categories with similarities were grouped into distinct, higher order conceptual themes.

EMERGING THEMES

The seven themes illustrated in Figure 7.1 emerged from the analysis of the data, representing the essential components of a group contract. A discussion of the set follows.

FIGURE 7.1. Emerging Themes of Group Contract and Analysis of Data

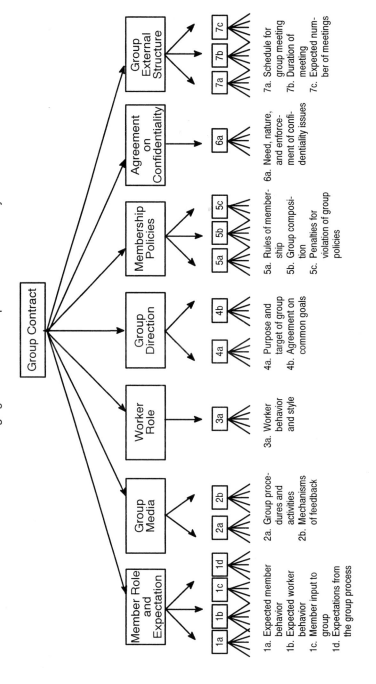

Member Role and Expectation

This category brought together all agreements and expectations among the group members regarding their role in the group. The members' expectations were from each other: "At times, each member will be expected to share parts of what she writes, with the group."* "I was thinking about group members needing to offer advice in a way that feels more like helping than attacking to the person receiving it."; expected inputs that *each member would give to the group*: "Two of them said they would be willing to help L. get in on conversations and in the group." "Participants in the group share a responsibility to one another to be involved with sessions on a regular basis since everyone's participation contributes to making this a productive experience."; and their expectations *from the group process*: "She would be able to start talking with people and be able to keep a conversation going." "He hoped to be able to make new relationships and would have a better picture of how he comes across." The pregroup interviews seemed to have created an extensive discussion among the members and the group worker regarding these member roles and expectations.

Group Media

This theme refers to the different activities, assignments and methods that the group would use to achieve its objectives. This included discussions and agreements about *group procedures and activities*: "I explained that we begin group with a check-in process of the week and move into a topic discussion."; and *mechanisms of feedback*: "Feedback from myself and other members should be given in a direct and supporting manner." "The facilitator will ask for written and confidential feedback from group members three separate times through the sixteen weeks."

Worker Role

This theme included the discussion of worker behavior and worker style. The theme refers more to the worker's description of her or his style of working and their role and behavior in the group. This is

---

*The examples used here are quoted from the group worker's pre-group interview.

different from the member expectations of the worker, which are more from the members' views. This category included all the *statements made by the worker regarding her or his role and behavior and style of working in the group*: "In facilitating this group, I will be providing some specific tasks and exercises for the group which will hopefully assist us in getting to know each other and determining what we can learn from each other." "In my work with groups, I strive to find a balance between promoting a supportive atmosphere while encouraging constructive challenging among members." "The only exception to this agreement would be in the event that I became aware that someone was in danger, in which case I would contact any individuals who I felt might be able to prevent harm from taking place." There was an attempt by the worker to reconcile any differences that existed between the member's expectation and the worker's understanding of the "worker role" in the group.

Group Direction

This theme brought together all discussion in the pregroup interview that revolved around the direction the group would take. This involved discussion about the purpose and target of the group: "Our general purpose will be to provide support and feedback to one another around the issues related to these children returning home who have been difficult to parent in the past." "I explain that the group was designed for women who had been arrested for domestic violence and who also needed a special focus placed on parenting issues."; and *agreement on common goals that the group would move toward achieving*: "I began by explaining that the purpose of a whole-group contract is to bring the individuals who make up the group together to form a unit." The analysis reveals a very conscious effort by the worker in attempting to achieve as much consensus as possible at this stage.

Membership Policies

This theme referred to discussions about the various policies that would apply to members in the group. This revolved around discussions about whether the group would be open or closed; *rules of membership*: "Members will be on time for meetings, will attend the group on a consistent basis, and intend to share at least one thought or feeling during each session." "Members of the group are expected to be on time and to bring the notebook that they are provided with on the first day." "Individuals who cannot attend a meeting should contact me at least twenty-four hours in advance." "Those who miss more than two meetings should arrange a time to meet with me individually to discuss whether this type of support service is appropriate for them at this time."; and group composition (age and type of other members): "Jane had a few questions about the number of women in the group."

Agreement on Confidentiality

This theme referred to the extensive discussion that took place between the members, and members and the worker, regarding the *need, nature, and the kind of enforcement to be made regarding member behavior and the penalties for violation of policies*: "Any violation of confidentiality will result in the removal of that person from the group." A large portion of the pregroup interviews revolved around *clarification of this confidentiality issue*: "I reiterated that they had all agreed to holding what was discussed in the group in confidence and that they had said they all wanted that and would respect it for each other." "I then went into detail about issues of confidentiality and the importance of creating a safe place to discuss issues. Mary M. had several questions about the issue of confidentiality so I spent a few minutes talking about it in detail."

Group External Structure

This theme brought together discussions and decisions made between the members and the worker regarding a schedule for the time of group meeting, the duration of the meeting, and the expected number of meetings for the entire group process.

These were the seven themes that surfaced as components of a group contract from the analysis of the data. Discussion among the worker and the group members around these themes appear focused on consensus making, in the way that Schopler and Galinsky cast consensus. They observed that group effectiveness is affected when

. . . there . . . [is] *sufficient consensus* on which goals the group will pursue. Sufficient consensus means that the group has enough support for particular goals to mobilize members. (Schopler and Galinsky, 1974, p. 140)

Achieving clarity and consensus regarding the reasons that members and worker are gathered as a group seems to appear, in the analyzed documents, as "the aim of the worker" and "the desire of the members." What, where, and how they will go about reaching goals was seen as instrumental in the agreed statements. The use of the themes would aid in this process of arriving at clarity and consensus on goals and instruments.

The use of the NUDIST program in analysis of narrative process records appears to sustain the potential of establishing a contract through a pregroup interview. At the same time, review of some contract terms is indicated. Earlier, nine terms were presented as having been culled from social group work literature. The contract term identified as #6 "choice and use of facilities" has never been mentioned by any worker, member, or prospective member—other than a worker's stating where a group meeting will occur—in over twenty-five years of testing this practice tool. While that would tend to indicate that the term is not likely to surface, the possibility of its emergence in the future cannot be eliminated. While "choice and use of facilities" is probably not a prominent issue in agreeing about service goals, it could appear. Issues might arise as to who would make the decisions about facilities, who would agree or need to agree, and what changes in facilities might need to be made and under what conditions these matters would be addressed.

In the present analysis, the concept of the group as a whole as a unit of reference did not emerge and may have to be examined more closely and repeatedly to determine whether it ought to be retained. The lack of its mention may be a function of the fact that the data analyzed came from the first meeting of prospective member and worker and the "we" character implied by "group as a whole" would not be operative.

This analysis and results seem to portend well for future knowledge-building ventures. NUDIST is a promising tool, as it makes possible a method of inquiry not previously available.

Future study of the promise of the findings in this analysis is certainly indicated. Study needs to be undertaken regarding which contract term/theme or terms/themes carry more of the load in the (sufficient) consensus which has the power to mobilize member and worker energy toward a goal. Study in that direction would tend to dictate a different model of analysis; perhaps one more quantitative than qualitative.

In addition, workers might use NUDIST to search the content of pregroup interviews for hidden agendas, subliminal intentions, or unavowed and covert goals of prospective members, and make those explicit and overt in full group meetings. Workers and researchers might identify which themes or terms contribute (and if so, with what frequency) to the consensus, and pair that finding with future research on the link between contract term agreements and members' perceptions of goal achievement.

More study needs to be addressed to detecting themes other than those the literature has presented. Perhaps the terms or themes, as they are presently known, need to be broken apart and their constituent parts examined for deeper or fuller significance. Perhaps themes or terms should be combined and new connotations of meaning explored. Just as in the case of the analysis here reported, in which shadings of what originally appeared as finite concepts could be recast as a similar but not identical term, future work might produce new syntheses of ideas. Evidence is not present to say with confidence that the *seven* themes which emerged from the analysis of practical application of the material found in the theoretical literature are the conceptual equivalents of the *nine* contract terms originally proposed. The subject begs for deeper investigation.

Do we know, from this report, whether the identified themes constitute the sufficient consensus which Schopler and Galinsky held out as energy mobilizing? No. But, we do have a tool to use in clarifying the matters which bear on beginning with groups. Without a doubt, investigation needs to be focused on whether and how the clarity, specificity, and explicitness of contract terms (or themes) connect themselves to goal achievement. And that will move the building of social group work knowledge one more important step forward.

REFERENCES

Cartwright D. and Zander, A. (Eds.) (1960). *Group Dynamics Research and Theory,* Second Edition. Evanston, IL: Row, Peterson.

Estes, R.J. and Henry, S. (1976). The therapeutic contract in work with groups: A formal analysis. *Social Service Review, 50*(4), 611-622.

Garvin, C. (1969). Complementarity in role expectations in groups: The member-worker contract. In Selected Papers, 96th Annual Forum, National Conference on Social Welfare, Emanuel Berlatsky (Ed.), 1969. New York: Columbia University Press, 127-145.

Hartford, M.E. (1966). Changing approaches in practice theory and techniques. In *Trends in Social Work Practice and Knowledge: NASW Tenth Anniversary Symposium.* New York: National Association of Social Workers.

Hartford, M.E. (1972). *Groups in Social Work.* New York: Columbia University Press.

Henry, S. (1972). *Contracted Group Goals and Group Goal Achievement.* Unpublished doctoral dissertation, University of Denver.

Henry, S. (1974, October). Use of contracts in social work with groups. Paper presented at the School of Applied Social Sciences Alumni Association Symposium, Cleveland, OH.

Henry, S. (1981). *Group Skills in Social Work.* Itasca, IL: F.E. Peacock Publishers.

Henry, S. (1992). *Group Skills in Social Work,* Second Edition. Belmont, CA: Wadsworth, Inc., Brooks/Cole Publishing Co.

Mills, T.M. (1967). *The Sociology of Small Groups.* Englewood Cliffs, NJ: Prentice-Hall.

Schopler, J. and Galinsky, M. (1974). Goals in social group work practice: Formulation, implementation, evaluation. In P. Glasser, R. Sarri, and R. Vinter (Eds.), *Individual Change Through Small Groups* (pp. 126-148). New York: Free Press.

Schwartz, W. (1962). Toward a strategy of group work practice. *Social Service Review, 36*(3), 268-279.

Chapter 8

Rebuilding a Divided Community Through the Use of Marathon Groups

Lourencia Hofmeyr

INTRODUCTION

The honeymoon for a new democratic South Africa is over. The reality of rebuilding the country with its tremendous problems, as well as its potential and opportunities, is dawning upon us. We will have to live up to this challenge.

In South Africa, the new welfare policy concentrates extensively on primary social care to provide basic services to the disadvantaged masses. In the light of this new and relatively unknown situation, procedures should be sought that can be time-effective as well as cost-effective, so that therapeutic services can be retained as far as possible, and also extended. In this, the use of marathon groups is a decided possibility and there is now a renewed interest in them.

HISTORICAL PERSPECTIVE ON MARATHON GROUPS

In 1963, a Dr. Lehner of the UCLA conducted a sensitivity laboratory for professionals and business executives that Fred Stoller (among others) attended. Out of this experience came an appreciation for group interaction that continued beyond the time parameters of traditional forms of group experience (Fullmer, 1971, p. 232). Marathon groups were first devised by George Bach and Fred Stoller in 1964 as a way of helping people, as Gladding (1991, p. 17) puts it, to become more authentically in touch with themselves. In 1967, Bach described the power of and the need for group marathons. Many other types of groups, such as encounter groups, sensory awareness groups, growth groups, and minithons also emerged during this period in which, according to Gladding (1991, p. 9), ". . . there was a group for everyone and everyone was in a group."

Psychotherapy was influenced by the sensitivity training field and its frequent use of intensive residential workshops in which the participants live together and meet in groups for several hours daily over several days (Yalom, 1975, p. 279). Social work with groups was of course not untouched by all this and the idea of extended groups became more established throughout the group work field.

In spite of the fact that the first marathon groups were already been established so long ago, there is still comparatively little information on this type of group available in social work literature. It seems as if, by far, most of the information comes from articles on group psychotherapy. This is also the case in the Republic of South Africa. Perhaps this is a good time to look at marathon groups with renewed interest.

POSSIBILITIES FOR UTILIZATION OF MARATHON GROUPS

It seems as if there are plenty of opportunities in which marathon groups can be utilized. In literature on group psychotherapy a wide variety of marathons is described. To mention but a few: marathon groups for alcoholics (Mintz, 1971, p. 352); for isolated college students (Berlin and Dies, 1974); for female narcotic addicts (Kilmann, 1974); for psychopaths (Raath, 1979); for drug users (Page, 1983); for incest offenders (Frey, 1987); for divorce adjustment (Byrne and Overline, 1991); and for individuals in groups and marriages to resolve conflict ". . . by learning to fight fairly" (Gladding 1991, p. 10). Drower (1993) describes an encounter weekend for women which was held in South Africa to facilitate interracial contact and understanding. In connection with disasters and terrifying events, Terr (1992) mentions an interesting number of possibilities. He points out that aid can be rendered through mini-marathon groups to, among other things, victims of hostage dramas, after civilian disasters, earthquakes and similar experiences. He also mentions the possibility of preparing professionals through mini-marathons to lead this type of group on their own.

In South Africa, marathon groups were successfully conducted in social work settings by undergraduate social work students of the University of Pretoria among adolescent boys in substitute care (Raath, 1988); with prisoners (Department of Correctional Services, 1990-1996); with primary school children who were struggling to cope with their parents' divorce and with multicultural high school pupils who have not been in the same school for a long time. The Kegotsamo parent guidance group, consisting of black domestic workers, was also conducted by a social work student (Christian Social Council (CSC) Report 1996); and with disadvantaged adolescents at high risk, and disadvantaged women who were helped to cope better with their circumstances (Pretoria Child and Family Care Society Report, 1996).

With less money available for welfare services in South Africa, and a vast number of disadvantaged people, every possible opportunity to get the work done should be considered. There should be an openness for innovative and creative ways to reach out and help people. With regard to traumatic experiences, killings, road accidents, hijacking of cars, and a high crime rate, the mini-marathon model of Terr (1992) after disasters, deserves consideration.

In a community where the differences between people had long been emphasized, social work with groups can play a vital role in the rebuilding process. Marathon groups can be used advantageously to help many people become more in touch with themselves and with others. The intrinsic qualities of such groups can possibly contribute toward bridging the vast gaps between the different cultures and enabling people to risk it with each other. Multicultural groups may perhaps benefit from the time-extended period, and experimentation with it seems to be important.

DESCRIPTION OF MARATHON GROUPS

Terms such as "marathon group," "encounter group," "marathon encounter group," and "time-extended group" are often used indiscriminately and interchangeably in literature. Time-extended group therapy has been used in clinical practice in several different formats. Definitions are thus sometimes drawn up from different perspectives and angles. Although the definitions may in broad terms sound alike, the content and methods used by the various approaches may be totally different. Length of duration, goals, and structuring can be different. The fact that aid-rendering within a marathon group does not require a specific theoretical perspective, makes it logical that different content may be given to the same words.

Guinan, Foulds, and Wright (1973, p. 177) point out that a marathon group is a technique in so far as it is a formally structured setting with which therapeutic changes are fostered and developed. Mintz (1971, p. 1) defines a marathon group as an island in time. She claims that it is a group of people who remains in continuous involvement with one another for a prolonged period of time, typically at least twenty-four hours. Marathon groups can be seen as an attempt to overcome certain problems which are experienced in conventional groups such as discontinuity, unsuccessful work-through of emotions, and difficulties establishing group cohesion.

GOALS OF MARATHON GROUPS

The purpose of marathon groups differs a great deal. In group psychotherapy literature some authors emphasize the growth aspect (Mintz, 1971, p. 6; Fullmer, 1971, p. 191). Authors differ on the treatment component of the marathon. Fullmer (1971, pp. 233, 235) does not see the marathon as a treatment form but as an experiential learning unit. He places a strong emphasis on self-exploration and fostering of personal responsibility while Allen (1990, pp. 368-371) and Gebhart and Grover (1974, p. 223) perceive it as a treatment form.

As the emphasis in social work with groups lies very much on promoting the social functioning and societal conditions of group members, this should be an important consideration when the goals of the group are defined. Students at the University of Pretoria emphasized the fact that the goals should be realistic and attainable in terms of time. Where therapeutic help cannot be offered sufficiently, the goal should rather be more didactic or growth-oriented.

Ample time should be available for personal attention to group members. The needs and potential of the group should be taken into account (CSC Report, 1996).

The purpose of the group must be clearly defined in the workers' own mind before the initial meetings, even though, according to Brandler and Roman (1991, p. 106), they recognize that the purpose will evolve with the clients' input and their expression of needs. Purposeful contact with group members during the preparation phase will prevent the worker from determining it by himself. Goals may be redefined. The goals and objectives of the group should be clear to all parties involved.

When the ideal of matching the goals of the group with the needs of the members is taken into account, the group categorization can be educational, growth, remedial, or socialization (Cf. Toseland and Rivas, 1984, pp. 19-26).

SOME CHARACTERISTICS OF MARATHON GROUPS

Extended Time

One of the major characteristics of the marathon is that extended time is spent together. Considerable variations occur in terms of what is meant by extended time. In broad terms, marathon groups are held over a few days or over a weekend and encompass long hours of treatment. The time span can differ between three-hour sessions in the case of a mini-marathon, but can be extended over three days with each session on the following day as part of ongoing group therapy sessions (Allen, 1990, p. 368); to nine-hour sessions which Mintz (1971, p. 237) refers to as mini-marathons. Yalom (1975, p. 278) refers to sixteen-hour marathons. Gebhart and Grover (1974, p. 223) prefer a twenty-four hour, nonstop treatment group. It thus seems as if everybody has his or her own preference. Some therapists allow little or no time for sleep and others do make provision for it. Different approaches to therapy have their own likes and dislikes, such as the Rogerians who prefer marathons under twelve hours (Gladding 1991, p. 53) while rational-emotive groups are conducted on a twelve- to thirty-six-hour basis, depending on the leader and the setting (Gladding, 1991, p. 68). Kilmann and Sotile (1976, p. 828) come to the conclusion (after researching marathon groups) that the existing data cannot resolve the issue of which of the following formats is most effective in producing desired change:

1. Continuous marathon format with no interruptions
2. A format that includes breaks for eating and/or sleeping
3. A format that is spaced over a number of days

Age, level of development, and attention span may be some of the criteria for determining the length of sessions.

Experience in terms of marathon groups in South Africa makes it clear that it is cheaper and more time-effective for the members and the group worker to go to a place once or twice for a long period, instead of on many different occasions for a short time (CSC Report, 1996). In the Kegotsamo (which means "rest a while") group, it was found practical for domestic workers to attend time-extended groups on successive Saturdays, as they did not have time during the week to attend long sessions. It also showed that if the needs of the group and its goals can be matched with longer sessions, it can be very useful. As Allen (1990, p. 369) points out, an extended session often develops "momentum," so the group progresses more rapidly, and members get to know and trust one another faster. Trust results in more openness, sharing, and cohesiveness—all of which are essential to the group therapeutic process. The same author also claims that in a newly formed group, cohesiveness, intimacy, and mutual trust develop more rapidly in an extended session in contrast to the usual group sessions, in which several months may be needed before strong emotions are expressed and intense relatedness develops. After an interlude, such as a vacation, an extended session tends to speed up the movement of the whole group and get things going. According to Allen (1990, p. 369) an extended session also can help to assimilate a new member or members into an ongoing group.

According to research done at the University of Pretoria (CSC Report, 1996 and Pretoria Child and Family Care Society Report, 1996) progress was more rapid in marathon sessions. Members seemed to be more involved and dependent on each other. Due to time pressure, discussions were more intense and focused. Both students and group members were aware of the fact that the whole process would be completed within two days and devoted themselves more wholeheartedly. Time was used to the utmost. It seemed as if the therapeutic atmosphere put positive pressure on members to get more involved in the process, thus contributing toward progress. Less time is needed for warm-up exercises and functional aspects during group meetings.

There was, however, a negative side to the time-extended nature of marathon groups in the sense that some students felt that too much had to be done in too little time. Some experienced that the limited time prevented real therapeutic aid rendering. Needs and problems of group members (which in ordinary group work could be handled during further meetings) sometimes got lost during marathon sessions. As pointed out, the goals should sometimes be changed. Furthermore, students were not always sure how to handle these aspects, and supervision was not as readily available as with traditional group work (CSD Report, 1996). Supervision should be available during breaks. Live supervision could also be considered during sessions.

It was also clear that, as in the case of children of divorced parents, the expectation of what type of aid could actually be given was sometimes more than what was possible during the duration of the marathon group. Students also experienced great difficulty in adjusting their planning and functional aids when it appeared necessary (CSD Report, 1996). Although some of the aspects with which undergraduate students had problems were related to their inexperience, this should nevertheless be taken into consideration when working with these types of groups. Possibilities to follow up group members—when necessary—are suggested by Gebhart and Grover (1974, p. 236) and Allen (1990, p. 370), to deal with unresolved or new issues. The possibility for further help for group members should also be available, and indeed this materialized in quite a few cases in the organizations where the students worked. Recontracting to form a new group is another possibility which should be kept in mind.

It seems that in marathon groups the members are often more inclined to turn to happenings in the group and to use them and not to withdraw. All this makes this type of group worthy of exploration. Continuous feedback, a great deal of interdependence, openness, sincerity, and development of insight makes marathons preeminently appropriate in South Africa's present situation.

Fatigue

Closely related to the length of marathon groups is the question of fatigue. According to Gladding (1991, p. 17), fatigue leads to a breakdown in participants' defenses, and an increase in their truthfulness. Allen (1990, p. 368) claims that with a longer meeting, fatigue often occurs in members, resulting in reduced defenses, less role-playing (lowering of inhibitions), and less concern about one's image. This often results in more genuineness, openness, and closeness with fellow members. Breakthroughs and insight may then be achieved.

In social work with groups this fatigue can be useful to a certain extent, but this matter should be regarded with the greatest care. Where eight group sessions were held within a period of two days, it was found that both students of the University of Pretoria and group members (especially children and adolescents) were exhausted by the fourth session. They recommended that no more than four sessions should be held, with ample time—especially for children's groups—to relax and play and to have some time for meals (CSC Report, 1996). In adolescent groups it is important to avoid the weakening of defenses by fatigue. He suggests frequent rest periods, as well as a full eight-hour break for sleep. Another possibility is to conduct sessions (over three to four successive days) for shorter periods. One or more marathon sessions could also be used in addition to the weekly group sessions to enhance the group involvement and potential for growth (Gazda, 1982, p. 130).

In South Africa, it may nevertheless be a useful way of dealing with long-standing problems to make use of the fact that in these groups there is talk of lowered defense mechanisms and accelerated interaction. Group workers should determine how much fatigue is appropriate. This will have consequences in terms of time needed. It will be worthwhile to experiment with marathon groups—in terms of cross-cultural groups where people have grown up in separate worlds—to see whether the discussions are not more relevant, intimate, intense, and purposeful. (Cf. Drower [1993] in this regard.)

STAGES IN MARATHON GROUPS

Four different stages are defined in group psychology literature on marathon groups. Raath (1979, p. 39), for example, distinguishes an initial, hostile, dependent, and terminal stage. This corresponds very well with the four stages of Northen (1988, pp. 185-332) namely an orientation-inclusion stage, a dissatisfaction and power conflict stage, a mutuality and work stage, and a separation, termination, and transition stage. The way in which the group is conducted in these stages may differ, but there are also similarities. Social work groups may also be more structured than encounter marathons.

In the *initial* stage, fears and fantasies occur about what might happen in the extended session, as well as issues of trust (Allen, 1990, p. 370). In this stage, pupils of the multicultural high school group, for example, were uneasy, and hardly spoke to each other (CSC Report, 1996). These issues must be recognized and worked through in both psychotherapy and social work groups before meaningful progress can be accomplished. Contracting or recontracting is necessary, rules must be explained, and goals should be defined. Structured experiences can also be used in social work groups, but must be selected in terms of their usability and acceptability within social work, and in a particular culture and setting. (Cf. Anderson, 1980, pp. 51-59 in this regard.)

In the *hostile* stage, the task of the group is to express emotions. Allen (1990, p. 370) points out the importance of enacting and working through conflicts of the past and the present, to achieve greater self-acceptance, relatedness, and authenticity in communication, and to deal with the issues of independence and interdependence present in group membership. This complies in broad terms with the dissatisfaction and power conflict stage. Social work with groups will handle this by understanding the group, strengthening relationships, enhancing positive motivation, clarifying purpose, stabilizing membership, influencing status and roles, resolving conflict, and working beyond the group (Northen, 1988, pp. 224-257). Social work groups should be true to their own methods and strategies in handling this stage.

In the *dependent* stage, (mutuality and work state) cohesion and intimacy are clear and group members get the most out of the group, whether it be in different ways in the different types of groups. By getting to know each other and being close to each other (they had to lead one another blindfoldedly) high school pupils from different cultures bridged the distance and experienced a close bond during this stage (CSC Report, 1996).

Gebhart and Grover (1974, p. 226) point out that members in the *terminal* stage begin to take responsibility for the need to achieve closure. They are more in touch with their feelings. This is also the case in social work groups. Separation, anxiety, and feelings of grief and loss are present. Loose ends must be wrapped up and be dealt with from a social work perspective. (Cf. Brandler and Roman, 1991, pp. 75-102.)

THE WORKER(S) IN MARATHON GROUPS

A group worker conducting marathon sessions must be able to take the pressure of a long, intense group session. Physical vitality and emotional well-being are important aspects of the make-up of marathon group workers. Gebhart and Grover (1974, p. 228) point out that such workers should be able to recognize and cope with their personal needs. Terr (1992, p. 85) states that a professional should not take the demanding role of a mini-marathon leader if he or she is, in the event of a disaster, too traumatized to see beyond personal concerns.

Various authors point out that a co-leader or co-worker is necessary and helpful in conducting marathon groups. Gebhart and Grover (1974, p. 229) are even of the opinion that marathons should always have a co-leader. They claim that co-leadership allows for more flexibility in stepping back from the group and expanding the leadership repertoire. Allen (1990, p. 370) points out that a cotherapist can observe what is happening from a different perspective and can contribute toward combating fatigue. A co-worker should be someone with whom the group worker has worked on other occasions, and someone with whom he or she feels comfortable.

Two workers can be a hindrance in using marathon social work groups in South Africa, as it makes the service more expensive, yet the advantages of using two workers can make the costs involved worthwhile.

ISSUES RELATED TO MARATHON GROUPS

Good preparation is of vital importance when working with marathon groups. Members and the group worker should be prepared for the extended time spent in the group and the whole process that awaits them. The worker should also, as far as possible, be thoroughly emotionally and functionally prepared. The functional preparation should, however, be flexible and adaptable. Especially for children's groups, but also for other groups, functional aids should be available when needed.

Also in terms of reporting, special needs exist when working with marathon groups. Little time is available for writing reports. See Appendix for an example of an abridged process report. It proved to work well during group work sessions conducted by students of the University of Pretoria.

THE VALUE OF MARATHON GROUPS
FOR SOCIAL WORK WITH GROUPS

The question of how useful marathon groups are is important. Of particular interest is whether participants experience lasting changes in their personal or interpersonal functioning. (Cf. Also Greenberg, Seeman, and Cassius, 1978, p. 66.)

Yalom (1975, pp. 280-281) points out that "(t)he results of marathon group therapy reported in the mass media and in scientific journals have boggled the mind." He remarks that the results are entirely based on anecdotal reports of various participants or questionnaires distributed shortly after the end of the meeting when there is strong group pressure. He concludes that no evidence exists to document the many extravagant claims. Kilmann and Sotile (1976, p. 847) have also questioned the research procedures of many of the evaluations on marathon groups and come to the conclusion that the overall findings do not provide support for general positive effects. Yalom (1975, p. 284) questions whether the marathon group precludes the use of long-term therapy, but does not deny its impact.

Although marathon groups are by no means a panacea or a crash program to change a society overnight, they have been very useful in South Africa so far. We have had, however, only limited experience with these groups. Especially among welfare organizations where the resources of money and time are scarce, marathon groups seem very useful. Not such an urgent demand occurs for marathon groups in institutions where people still have to attend group work meetings, and money and transport do not create such a big problem. Marathon groupwork might also be very useful in rural areas where welfare services are scarce. Perhaps we will also be able to reach new client populations. Patients waiting for mobile medical services may be, for example, a potential target group.

Less funds are now available in South Africa to support the participation of welfare organizations in the training of student social workers. Marathon groups can be used to keep costs low for such training. This seems a feasible way to involve welfare organizations in social work education, particularly as students and faculty learn to use marathon groups for training purposes. Marathon groups will have to be used to keep cost and time factors for welfare organizations as low as possible, while still offering good training and aid.

CONCLUSION

We still lack a great deal of knowledge regarding marathon group therapy. We need to have a sound theoretical base for this therapy and to know more about its use. We also need information on the response of specific types of groups to marathon groups. We need to know more about the ideal length of the meetings as a whole and about marketing this approach. Little is known about how we can use this therapy for improved relations among the different cultures in South Africa, and how it can assist in situations where people have to learn rapidly how to co-exist with one another. Nevertheless, experimentation with marathon group therapy seems to be worthwhile. Perhaps we can rebuild a divided community in this way.

Appendix

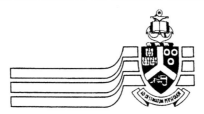

ABRIDGED PROCESS REPORT
AND EVALUATION OF A MARATHON GROUP

(This report must be completed after the termination of every meeting.)

1. Name of student: _____

2. Number of meeting: _____ 3. Date: _____

4. Venue: _____ 5. Duration: _____

6. Membership: Present: _____ Absent: _____

7. Subject of the group discussion: _____
_____

8. Goals: _____
_____

9. Objectives: _____
_____
_____
_____
_____

10. Preparation:
10.1 Functional: _____
_____

10.2 Emotional: _____
_____

11. The group process:

Rating scale:
1 = Very poor   *3 = Average*   *5 = Very good*
2 = Poor   *4 = Good*

		1	2	3	4	5	Remarks
11.1	Group motivation						
11.2	Control						
11.3	Atmosphere						
11.4	Group cohesion						
11.5	Program planning						
11.6	Relationships						
11.7	Values and norms						
11.8	Structuring						

12. Skills of the group worker:

		1	2	3	4	5	Remarks
12.1	Purposeful implementation of the principles						
12.2	Building significant relationships						
12.3	Understanding and handling of group feelings						
12.4	Identification and handling of the group process						
12.5	Programming						
12.6	Observation						
12.7	Communication						
12.8	Conducting group discussion						
12.9	Exploration						
12.10	Utilization of functional aids						
12.11	Utilization of co-group worker						

13. Forms of aid-rendering:

13.1 Handling of feelings:

		1	2	3	4	5	Remarks
13.1.1	Support						
13.1.2	Handling of catharsis						
13.1.3	Focusing						
13.1.4	Reflection						
13.1.5	Handling of resistance						
13.1.6	Handling of conflict						
13.1.7	Handling of transference						

13.2 Direct influencing:

		1	2	3	4	5	Remarks
13.2.1	Information provided						
13.2.2	Advice						
13.2.3	Confirmation						

13.3 Increase of insight:

		1	2	3	4	5	Remarks
13.3.1	Clarification						
13.3.2	Interpretation						
13.3.3	Confrontation						
13.3.4	Projective exploration						

13.4 Attitudinal change:

		1	2	3	4	5	Remarks
13.4.1	Worker's inputs with regard to decision making						

13.5 Behavioral change:

		1	2	3	4	5	Remarks
13.5.1	Worker's inputs with regard to modeling						
13.5.2	Assistance to proceed to action						
13.5.3	Support for perseverance						

14. Phase of group:

Preparation	Start	Participation	Utilization	Termination

15. Schematic presentation of group interaction:

16. Evaluation of the success of the meeting:

		1	2	3	4	5	Remarks
16.1	Goal achievement						
16.2	Course						
16.3	Resources						
16.4	Reaction of group members						

17. Aspects for supervision:

17.1

17.2

17.3

_____

Signature of Student

_____

Date

REFERENCES

Allen, M.G. 1990. Using extended sessions in ongoing group therapy. *Psychiatric Annals, 20*(1): 368-371, January.

Anderson, J.D. 1980. Structured experiences in growth groups in social work. *Social Casework, 61*(5): 227-287, May.

Berlin, J.S. and Dies, R.R. 1974. Differential group structure: The effects on socially isolated college students. *Small Group Behavior, 5*(4): 462-472, November.

Brandler, S. and Roman, C.P. 1991. *Group Work: Skills and Strategies for Effective Interventions.* Binghamton, NY: The Haworth Press, Inc.

Byrne, R.C. and Overline, H.M. 1991. A study of divorce adjustment among para-professional group leaders and group participants. *Journal of Divorce and Remarriage, 17*(1/2): 171-191.

Christian Social Council. 1996. *Report on Student Unit for Practical Social Work Training for the University of Pretoria.* Pretoria.

Department of Correctional Services. 1990-1996. *Report on groupwork.*

Drower, S. 1993. The contribution of group work in a changing South Africa. *Social Work with Groups, 16*(3): 5-22.

Frey, C. 1987. Minimarathon group sessions with incest offenders. *Social Work, 32*(6): 534-535, November-December.

Fullmer, D.W. 1971. *Counseling: Group Theory and System.* Cranston, RI: The Carroll Press Publishers.

Gazda, G.M. (Ed.). 1982. *Basic Approaches to Group Psychotherapy and Group Counseling.* Springfield, IL: Thomas.

Gebhart, J.E. and Grover, E.C. 1974. The 24-hour marathon. *The Journal of Pastoral Care, 28*(4): 221-240.

Gladding, S.T. 1991. *Group Work: A Counseling Specialty.* New York: Macmillan Publishing Company.

Greenberg, H., Seeman, J. and Cassius, J. 1978. Personality changes in marathon therapy. *Psychotherapy: Theory, Research and Practice, 15*(1): 61-67. Spring.

Guinan, J.F., Foulds, M.L. and Wright, J.C. 1973. Do the changes last? A six-month follow-up of a marathon group. *Small Group Behavior, 4*(2): 177-180, May.

Kilmann, P.R. 1974. Marathon group therapy with female narcotic addicts. *Psychotherapy: Theory, Research and Practice, 11*(4): 339-342, Winter.

Kilmann, P.R. and Sotile, W.M. 1976. The marathon encounter group: A review of the outcome literature. *Psychological Bulletin, 83*(5): 827-850.

Mintz, E.E. 1971. *Marathon Groups, Reality and Symbol.* New York: Avon Books.

Northen, H. 1988. *Social Work with Groups,* Second Edition. New York: Columbia University Press.

Page, R.C. 1983. Marathon group counseling with illicit drug users: A study of the effects of two groups for 1 month. *Journal for Specialists in Group Work, 8*(3): 114-125, September.

Pretoria Child and Family Care Society. 1996. *Report on Student Unit for Practical Social Work Training for the University of Pretoria*. Pretoria.

Raath, E. 1988. *Marathon-groepwerk met Adolessente seuns in Substituutsorg, met die oog die verbetering van selfbeeld*. Fourth-year script. University of Pretoria, Pretoria.

Raath, H.A. 1979. *Die terapeutiese effek van Marathongroepe op die psigopaat*. Unpublished MA (Clinical Psychology) dissertation. University of South Africa, Pretoria.

Terr, L.C. 1992. Mini-marathon groups: Psychological "first aid" following disasters. *Bulletin of the Menniger Clinic, 56*(1): 76-86, Winter.

Toseland, R.W. and Rivas, R.F. 1984. *An Introduction to Group Work Practice*. New York: Macmillan Publishing Company.

Yalom, I. 1975. *The Theory and Practice of Group Psychotherapy*, Second Edition. New York: Basic Books.

Chapter 9

It's More Than a Plumbing Problem

Barbara Neilson

Surgery, invasive procedures, and examinations for pediatric urology patients often involve the external genitalia. These patients may also require repeated hospitalizations and frequent hospital clinic visits. For many years the psychosocial, sexual, and social development of these patients have not been viewed to be as crucial as surgical correction. The multidisciplinary team on the urology program at The Hospital for Sick Children (HSC) was created in response to improve team, patient, and family collaboration and communication which have brought to the forefront the importance of these issues.

A 1992 unpublished survey of seventy pediatric urology programs in North America, conducted by this author, demonstrated a shortage of programs addressing the psychological, sexual, and social needs of their patients and families. It has been noted extensively in the group work literature that populations that have common concerns and goals can be served very effectively through the use of groups (Northen, 1989). Pediatric urologic populations certainly meet this criteria, and our experience has been that groups are effective. I hope by the conclusion of this chapter that the reader will have an increased understanding of the complexities of the population served and the benefits that the group process has brought to building a supportive sense of community.

This chapter will highlight both innovative ideas and new developments through the use of groups with both the team and the patient and family populations. These interventions address the following: (1) recognition that urologic surgery and procedures can have a negative impact on a child's self-esteem and body image unless psychosocial issues are addressed; (2) recognition that this patient population frequently can be classified as having diagnoses that are either rare, and/or difficult to discuss, due to the nature of the surgery and procedures that are necessary.

Feelings of isolation are not uncommon for both parents and patients, and siblings. It is not rare for new and for some seasoned staff on the urology unit, to experience discomfort in talking with the patients and families about the intense feelings these conditions elicit. Group interventions include the following:

1. Group education for, and ongoing support of frontline team members to promote discussion of sexuality issues openly with patients and families. Recognition that sexuality of children is not an area with which many professional health care providers are comfortable.
2. The use of weekly parent support group meetings to address psychosocial, sexual, networking, and educational issues for parents of pediatric urology patients. These include both inpatient groups and outpatient waiting room groups.
3. An annual concurrent group day for bladder exstrophy patients and families.
4. The development of an Internet mailing list discussion group for families of children with bladder exstrophy.
5. Future directions that include the increased use of computer assisted groups, both closed and open-ended, for the provisions of support services to the pediatric urology population.

THE PATIENTS AND THEIR "WATERWORKS"

Examples of some of the diagnoses that are seen within the pediatric urology program at HSC include ambiguous genitalia, hypospadias, and bladder exstrophy.

Ambiguous Genitalia

"Ambiguous genitalia in children constitutes a group of disorders that are rare, but important. It is imperative that the precise cause be identified as quickly as possible so that the appropriate sex of rearing can be assigned. Any delay may result in death in early infancy from an uncorrected metabolic disorder, the appearance of inappropriate secondary sexual changes at puberty, or malignant degeneration of the gonads at puberty" (Aaronson, 1992, p. 977). The cause of intersexuality is frequently based on hormonal conditions during the fetal development. Sometimes metabolic or chromosomal anomalies play a part. Whatever the cause, most parents hear of the condition of intersex for the first time when they are told that their child has it.

Hypospadias

A newborn may present with ambiguous genitalia. Gender assignment is the first challenge for parents and the medical team. If male gender is assigned, a hypospadias condition will need to be addressed. Penoscrotal hypospadias is the most severe form of this congenital defect of the penis, resulting in the incomplete development of the urethra. In this condition, the abnormal meatus opens into the perineum. Put simply, boys with this unrepaired condition urinate from an opening at the base of their penis. Chordee (an abnormal curvature of the penis) is an associated anomaly. Nine percent of these patients have undescended testes and inguinal hernias or hydroceles (Duckett, 1990). The initial surgery is generally scheduled at around twelve months of age. For the more severe forms of hypospadias, a staged repair is planned.

Bladder Exstrophy

"Exstrophy of the bladder is part of a spectrum of anomalies involving the urinary and genital tracts, the musculosketal system, and sometimes the intestinal tract. Most anomalies are related to defects of the abdominal wall, bladder, genitalia, pelvic bones, rectum, and anus" (Gearhart, 1992, p. 579). Initial surgical correction occurs at twenty-four to seventy-two hours of age, and entails the child being placed in Gallows traction for a period of two to three weeks. A minimum of two further surgeries will occur over the next few years.

Some of the secondary medical conditions that attend with these disorders are: (1) incontinence; (2) reflux; (3) urinary tract infections; (4) dysfunctional voiding. All of these diagnoses may require surgical correction. In recent years, many advances in surgical techniques have greatly improved the surgical outcome for these patients. Alongside the surgical advances, there has been a growth in the multidisciplinary team involvement in the patient's care. Recognition has occurred among the multidisciplinary team members that patients and families are dealing with many issues that are either not solved immediately or will never be solved by surgical correction. The stresses that we have identified are numerous and include:

- Repeated hospitalizations and surgeries
- Trauma caused by repeated procedures and surgeries on one of the most private areas of the child's body, genitals
- Uncertainty about the final outcome of the repeated surgeries
- Recognition that the surgical "fix," will most likely not leave the child looking "normal"
- Uncertainty about future sexuality, sexual function and fertility, and many parents feeling uncomfortable about addressing such questions unless directly given the opportunity and permission
- Teasing by peers

For example, these children have to contend with having to wear diapers, catheterizations, or, as young boys, having to sit on the toilet to urinate instead of standing. Teasing from classmates for any of these problems is very common, even in children of kindergarten age.

THE MULTIDISCIPLINARY HEALTH CARE TEAM

The need to address issues of sexuality with a group of patients on the urology unit was identified by staff nurses who were concerned about their ability to provide appropriate nursing interventions for pediatric patients. The questions and behavior of preadolescent and adolescent patients were instrumental in bringing together the multidisciplinary group to address patient and family sexuality issues. In 1989 this author was assigned to the pediatric urology unit in a .4 FTE capacity as a clinical social worker. Other than various nursing staff, the multidisciplinary team included a child life specialist, consulting psychiatrist, and input from the urologists on the service.

The team identified (through discussions with the staff nurses) that it was difficult to be proactive in discussing the needs and the concerns of both the patients and the parents, when staff themselves were not comfortable discussing issues of sexuality. The team decided that weekly rounds would begin that would be both educational and supportive of staff who were dealing with issues of sexuality with this patient population.

Strategies included talking about sexuality and issues that had arisen with various patients as well as staff's general discomfort with the issues. As we explored the issues, it was apparent that a number of the adolescent male patients were trying out their sexuality and ability to relate to the opposite sex with the nurses. This had caused much discomfort among the staff, who did not know how to respond to some of the overtures. Within the group context, as staff began to feel that they could trust one another, it was possible to reframe this behavior to that of adolescents feeling comfortable with nurses from whom they had nothing to hide.

These patients had often spent their early childhood and adolescent years hiding conditions from friends and in some cases, families. They did not know how to approach members of the opposite sex, but were aware that the nurses knew everything there was to know about their physical condition, and therefore felt somewhat freer to try out these behaviors. Within the group context we were able to begin to role-play some of these situations to give staff the tools to respond in a helpful manner. This meant that they could interpret some of the behavior, redirect it, and begin a dialogue about patients' feelings about themselves. The cohesion in the nursing group grew as they became more comfortable in behaving in a proactive manner with their patients, in beginning to identify issues sooner and to be able to provide interventions that were helpful to the patients. Through these discussions it also became more apparent who the patients were who needed to be referred to the author and/or the consulting psychiatrist.

The indicators of a well-functioning group became more apparent, in that the staff group that was meeting shared a sense of purpose, the development of mutual acceptance, and a growing understanding of the complementary nature of their roles. Although the urologists consulted in regard to the medical and surgical needs of patients they did not attend the multidisciplinary sexuality rounds. The cohesion that was growing among other health care providers in their ideas about providing service to these patients was increasing but was not equally shared by the surgeons. Surgeons have not historically availed themselves of psychosocial supports and resources for their patients (Pharis and Eisler, 1990).

The surgeons are basically involved with performing surgery or running very busy clinics which made it difficult if not impossible for them to attend the sexuality rounds. This author and key nursing staff found other ways to promote the change in practice that was occurring in the program with individual urologists at every possible opportunity. Through the sexuality rounds group we were able to begin to identify some of the basic needs of the patients and families for information. These issues were identified and shared with the surgeons. Some of the questions were as follows:

From parents:

• Is my child a girl or a boy?
• What do I tell my family and friends?
• What shall I name my child?
• Will my son ever be able to have intercourse? Will he be fertile? How many surgeries will he have?

From children/adolescents:

• I'm a boy, but I have a hole.
• Is it ever going to look normal?
• My penis looks like a cauliflower.
• Why doesn't the doctor just cut it off? Who would ever want me looking like this?
• Steven Spielberg couldn't have done as good a job.
• Why do I have to sit to pee, when other boys stand up?

In meetings with increasing numbers of parents and patients it was clear that feelings of isolation and feelings of differentness were common. Many of the patients had diagnoses of rare disorders and frequently we found that many had never met anyone with conditions similar to those or to others who were struggling with some of the same psychosocial issues. The idea of mutual support groups with parents and families of children with a chronic condition is not new and has resurfaced repeatedly (Leff and Walizer, 1992). It was clear that psychoeducational and informational groups as well as support groups could be very useful for these families.

IMPLEMENTATION OF STRATEGIES TO MEET IDENTIFIED NEEDS

The development of groups beyond the initial multidisciplinary team has been an ongoing and dynamic process. Initially, the focus was on two specific groups. One was a weekly parent coffee hour for parents of inpatients; another was a bladder exstrophy concurrent group day. Later, two groups now in their infancy were developed: an outpatient clinic waiting-room group and an Internet mailing-list group.

The Parent Group

By starting a weekly parent coffee hour we hoped to achieve the following:

- Help parents to manage the complexities of the hospital system
- Parent-to-parent sharing of supportive strategies
- Provision of community and hospital resource information
- Provision of a forum for feedback from parents in a supportive setting regarding their experience during hospitalization

Action Plan

Literature about success in establishing groups in hospital settings addresses the issue of needing to have stakeholders in agreement with the groups. In following this, the nurse manager and the program social worker conducted a survey of nursing staff on the unit and of the parents. The purpose of this was to determine if the idea would be supported by both groups. Mutual support was considered to be key to its success. The results of the two surveys showed positive support for the group by both staff and parents. These results were shared with the urologists. A letter was posted in the patients' rooms describing the group. On Wednesday morning unit rounds, the parents were reminded that the coffee hour would take place that day. An announcement was then made over the intercom at the commencement of the group and the co-leader quickly toured the unit encouraging parents to participate.

The group began with an introduction stating its rationale. We briefly discussed the need for a break from the children, a chance to meet other parents, and an opportunity to learn about the hospital and community resources. We also indicated that we wanted feedback from the parents about things that we did well and things that we needed to improve. Refreshments were served. The number of parents in attendance varied from one to five or six at a time.

Outcomes

Many parents who had previously attended the group made a point of coming back the next time they were in the hospital, even when they were situated on other units. Parents often expressed their lack of knowledge about the hospital and community resources that we described and utilized the information afterward to take advantage of resources. Parents shared with one another successful strategies for dealing with key frustrations. We introduced issues of sexuality and body image in the group in such a way that gave parents permission to talk about it. We then discovered that they were able to discuss some of their fears and were grateful to hear about resources that were available to them. When we did not mention sexuality, it was not discussed in the group. The use of permission-giving interventions appeared to be significant.

Conversation often turned to schooling, teasing, and behavioral issues. Intervention and management options were suggested both by the parents and the group leaders. The feedback that we were able to provide to staff helped them to view the coffee hour as useful for this particular group of parents. Some of the parents developed closer relationships with one another from the ward coffee hours and maintained contact on their own. They began to approach the author with requests for group support for their families and the children. They all expressed the feelings of isolation that they as parents as well as the children had experienced. With various genital anomalies, it is common for families not to discuss the condition outside of their own family system. They frequently shared feelings of shame as well as discomfort in talking with others. Many of the children had genitals that have an abnormal appearance, they may wear diapers, or they may need to use artificial diversions in order to eliminate both urine and/or feces.

The Bladder Extrophy Group Day

One of the affected groups mentioned at the beginning of this chapter was that of children born with bladder exstrophy. This group was identified as being in need of a chance for the patients and families to meet one another. It was felt that by offering a day to all family members a number of needs could be met. These include support, psychoeducation, and a chance for siblings to gain some understanding of the condition that is so time-consuming in their families. Through the idea of a family day that would run concurrent groups for parents, children, and siblings, we hoped to achieve the following:

- An opportunity for patients with a very rare disorder (1 in 40,000 to 50,000 live births) to obtain information and to meet others who are similarly affected
- An opportunity for families to discuss financial and emotional costs associated with many repeated hospitalizations and surgeries, the difficulties of living with a hidden condition (e.g., incontinence and invasive procedures), and an opportunity for patients and parents to discuss their concerns about psychosocial and sexual development. An opportunity for siblings to gain more knowledge of the condition and to gain a sense of belonging to a larger group

Development of the Group Day

We have now had the experience of running an exstrophy family day for three years. Initially a planning committee made up of social workers, bedside nurses, Clinical Nurse Specialist, Nurse Educator, Child Life Specialist, and parents was convened. Consultation with the psychiatrist and the urologists occurred regularly. Our planning included contacting other pediatric hospitals, and we were able to send a patient to another center to receive feedback. We were most fortunate to have a patient with bladder exstrophy who was now a resident psychiatrist. She brought a unique outlook to the process.

The resultant day included a mix of large and small group experiences for all participants. The parents' first workshop was a large group that listened to a panel of adult exstrophy patients discuss their own personal experiences. This provided an opportunity to hear of strategies that had helped these young adults, as well as affording an opportunity to ask questions that they had wondered about for years.

The afternoon workshops were small groups, and were designated by topic, e.g., building your child's self-esteem, medical issues, independence issues for adolescents, etc. Occurring at the same time were groups for children ages five to seven and eight to ten. Child care was provided for children younger than five.

The children's agenda included a tour of the operating room, tour of the microbiology lab, and an opportunity to develop questions with a nurse, to then ask the doctors. For many children this proved to be a first opportunity to ask questions without their parents. It is clear from the feedback that the family-to-family contact is a crucial component of providing care to this patient population.

Outpatient Clinic Waiting Room Group

With the amalgamation of the inpatient unit, and the trend toward shortened length of stay in the hospital following surgery, the writer developed an outpatient waiting-room group. The idea of a waiting room group has been discussed in the literature (Holmes-Garrett, 1989). The urology waiting room experience can be daunting. Each doctor has a clinic day on which forty-five to seventy-five patients may be booked. The waiting room is a converted playroom that can get quite crowded. The patient mix includes first-time patients, pre- or postoperative visits, and routine follow-up for chronic cases.

Goals for the waiting room group were similar to those of the inpatient group: education, support, empowerment, and feedback to assess ongoing needs of the patients and families. The group is scheduled for peak times in the clinic, and from the viewpoint of the rest of the team, it gives the parents something to focus on other than the wait.

The Internet Mailing List Group

The idea of computer-mediated groups is a newer innovation. (Weinberg et al., 1995). The patient population with a rare condition is a good match for a computer support group. The population is frequently spread out over a large geographic area, and this makes it difficult for potential members to meet. With this in mind, the writer has set up a mailing list support group for families and patients with bladder exstrophy. This is an open-ended, open membership type of group that has the potential to have members from around the world. The group has now been active for one year, and has thirty-five members. It has been exciting to watch the development of the group and to see the parallels with more conventional groups. Membership is being derived through postings on Usenet news groups, the pediatric urology list serve, the *Bladder Exstrophy Newsletter,* and word of mouth.

The positive aspects for this type of group are mutual support, education, and a lessened sense of isolation. One drawback is that the group may become too large for the type of discussion that could occur in a smaller group setting. Also, one does not really know the members in a way that is possible in a face-to-face group.

CONCLUSION

Any group leader who is involved with a patient population that has had to deal with a chronic and rare condition should find our experience useful. Patients and families have a need to explore their feelings and options about invasive and unpleasant treatments. They frequently are involved in a medical system that does not take these feelings into consideration and with professionals who are not comfortable with their own feelings about the issues with which the clients are struggling.

The following points are important for a group leader to consider in taking on such a population through the use of a group:

• Become comfortable and knowledgeable about the medical and surgical terminology and treatment plans affecting the group members.
• Develop a comfort level with proactively bringing up issues of sexuality both with the group, and with professionals dealing with group members.
• Recognize that a group can choose its own direction, but often needs permission to discuss taboo topics. If the leader can put people at ease initially, the group will develop its own comfort level with carrying through on the topics.
• Ensure that other health care professionals can have some direct feedback from group members about the usefulness of the group process. If possible, have the other professionals participate.

The community of pediatric urology patients and families has continued to show growing cohesion over the past eight years. The growth of the use of groups has played a major part in this development. Future plans include the use of a closed group on the computer for parents of children whose gender has been reassigned. This is a group who have wanted the support, but who have also been afraid of sharing their secret face to face. Other populations who are aware of our Internet support group have asked for a similar group to be started. Research in the area of outcomes and group development with the new technology has much potential.

In summary, the use of a group work framework has contributed to the growing sense of community for a population that has been overlooked in the past.

REFERENCES

Aaronson, I.A. (1992). Sexual differentiation and intersexuality. In P. Kelalis, L. King, and B. Belman (Eds.), *Clinical Pediatric Urology, Volume Two* (pp. 977-1014). Philadelphia, PA: W.B. Saunders Company.
Duckett, J. (1990). Hypospadias repair. In D. Frank and J.H. Johnston (Eds.), *Operative Pediatric Urology* (pp. 199-208). New York: Churchill Livingstone.

Gearhart, J.P. (1992). Bladder and urachal abnormalities: The exstrophy-epispadias complex. In P. Kelalis, L. King, and B. Belman (Eds.), *Clinical Pediatric Urology, Volume One* (pp. 579-618). Philadelphia, PA: W.B. Saunders Company.

Holmes-Garrett, C. (1989). The crisis of the forgotten family: A single session group in the ICU waiting room. *Social Work with Groups, 12*(4): 141-158.

Leff, P. and Walizer, E. (1992). The uncommon wisdom of parents at the moment of diagnosis. *Family Systems Medicine, 10*(2): 147-168.

Northen, H. (1989). Social work practice with groups in health care. *Social Work with Groups, 12*(4): 7-25.

Pharis, M.E. and Eisler, E. (1990). Psychological implications of childhood meatotomies. *Child and Adolescent Social Work, 7*(6): 461-474.

Weinberg, N., Schmale, J.D., Uken, J., and Wessel, K. (1995). Computer-mediated support groups. *Social Work with Groups, 17*(4): 43-54.

SECTION IV:
WORKSHOPS

Chapter 10

Group Work with Adolescent Immigrant Groups: Issues, Obstacles, and Principles

Roni Berger

ADOLESCENT IMMIGRANTS: REVIEW OF ISSUES

Adolescent immigrants are a high-risk population because they are caught simultaneously in a combined developmental and cultural transition that causes them to experience a unique build-up of stresses (Baptiste, 1990; Mirsky and Prawer, 1992).

Both immigration and adolescence are total, unstable, and stormy transitions that involve multiple losses. The combination sharpens the characteristic stresses of identity formation, belonging, and control over one's life (Grinberg and Grinberg, 1989). For adolescent immigrants these issues are more complicated because they lose stability, friends, school, culture, and country in a shaky phase of their life. The developmental and relocation-related effects exacerbate each other and the aforementioned issues become more severe and acute (Lee, 1988; Mirsky and Prawer, 1992; Goodenow and Espin, 1993).

Adolescent immigrants have limited resources to help them cope with these intensified needs. Several factors prevent their parents from providing support to their children. First, as distancing from parents is a typical aspect of the adolescents' struggle for autonomy, the adolescents are reluctant to turn to their parents for help. The typical parent-

The author is grateful to the staff of the Russian Adolescent Project (RAP) in the Jewish Board of Services for Families and Children (JBSFC) for their invaluable contribution to this chapter. Portions of this work originally appeared in the *Journal of Child and Adolescent Group Theory*, Vol. 6/No. 4, 1996, pp. 169-179. Reprinted with permission.

adolescent gap is widened by the anger many of the youngsters feel toward parents for imposing immigration on them (Landau, 1983; Gold, 1989) and by the fact that adolescents learn from the norms of the absorbing culture faster than their parents (Landau-Stanton, 1985; Baptiste, 1993). In addition, the parents themselves are experiencing the turmoil of immigration and struggles to find a job, address basic needs of the family, and adjust to the new culture. They are faced with rehabilitating their own sense of identity and belonging and, consequently, are not always available to provide the much-needed help.

Immigration cuts off the youngsters from the extra-familial sources of support, such as peers, extended family, schoolmates, and neighbors. Consequently adolescent immigrants are isolated, lack social connectedness, and need help.

Many immigrants are reluctant to use traditional mental health services. They are suspicious and cautious regarding authority and "establishment-related" counseling services. This reluctance stems from their original culture, which discourages sharing of feelings and self-disclosure outside the family, or from their experiences with the political abuse of services in their homeland (Goldstein, 1979). Programs that can address these unique issues are necessary. Group work is suggested as an effective modality to achieve this purpose. The next section of this chapter will discuss the advantages of group work in servicing adolescent immigrants.

WHY GROUP WORK IS A USEFUL MODALITY FOR HELPING ADOLESCENT IMMIGRANTS

Evidence regarding the effectiveness of group work with immigrants has been inconclusive. Group work is recognized as a useful modality in treating adolescents because of their general tendency to associate in groups (Leader, 1991; Henry, 1992). Glassman and Skolnik (1984) and Furnham and Bochner (1986) have presented clinical and empirical evidence about the usefulness of the group modality in servicing adolescent immigrants. Halberstadt and Mandel (1989) discussed the difficulties involved because self-disclosure and sharing of feelings with strangers are not acceptable in many of the immigrants' cultures of origin. However, the experience in the Jewish Board of Services for Families and Children is that a growing number of immigrants are participating in all kinds of groups (Berger, 1996).

Using group work with adolescent immigrants has several advantages. First, the group provides participants with a peer system that substitutes for friends and classmates lost to immigration. Adolescents prefer peers over adults as sources for support (Blos, 1979). Building on the age-appropriate preference for peer involvement, the group provides participants with an opportunity to belong to a social network and to share the experience of immigration with other adolescents who are going through a similar process. The peer group diminishes their isolation and validates their feelings of confusion, shame, anger, and frustration. In enables them to share experiences related to relocation—such as being rejected, ridiculed, and discriminated against—and to mourn losses. In the group, members realize that their difficulties are common to many adolescent immigrants and are caused by objective circumstances rather than by their own failure (Leader, 1991; Shulman, 1993). The "all-in-the-same-boat" phenomenon reduces the anxiety of group members, alleviates their feelings of pain, helplessness, guilt, anger, and frustration, and also helps them regain a sense of identity.

Second, the group offers participants an opportunity to acquire an understanding of American norms and to learn and rehearse in a safe environment social skills essential for living in the new culture. Mastery of social knowledge and skills helps group members gain a sense of control over their lives, raises their self-confidence, improves their acclimatization to the new culture and empowers them (Glassman and Skolnik, 1984; Furnham and Bochner, 1986).

The group may empower members by exposing them to adolescents who immigrated earlier and who can serve as powerful role models. Such encounters instill hope: "Here is somebody who knows from personal experience what I am going through, who was in the same situation and who has made it. Maybe I can also make it."

In spite of the advantages in addressing issues of adolescent immigrants, the use of groups may face several obstacles.

OBSTACLES TO EFFECTIVE GROUP WORK
WITH ADOLESCENT IMMIGRANTS

Several factors interfere with applying the modality of group work with immigrant adolescents. A major factor is parents' opposition to their children's participation in a group. One source of this attitude is the native cultural background. Many immigrants come from cultures that do not appreciate activity groups or therapy groups. Parents often see participation in groups as a "waste of time" and prefer that their children invest their time and effort in schoolwork rather than in social activities, the value of which they fail to recognize because "talking alone does not help." The negative outlook of parents toward groups is furthered by their anxiety that their children will "wash the family's dirty clothes in public," share information that the family would prefer to keep secret. Since the parents feel very insecure in the new society, the prospect of strangers learning about their private matters is scary to them; they refuse to give permission for their children to take part in activities that may call for sharing information.

Even though most adolescents adjust to the new culture and adopt its norms faster than their parents, the norms of their cultures of origin that emphasize protection of privacy and reject self-disclosure as inappropriate, may affect their readiness to participate in a group.

An additional obstacle is the attitude of immigrants from certain cultures toward groups. For example, immigrants from the former Soviet Union are familiar with the group modality because groups were a major component in the Soviet culture. However, the idea of group activities carries negative associations for them. Self-disclosure and sharing of feelings are not acceptable in the Russian culture, and were dangerous under the Soviet regime (Halberstadt and Mandel, 1989). This combination of negative experience and cultural reservations yields an ambivalent attitude toward groups (Berger, 1996). In some South American and Far Eastern cultures, the extended family rather than the peer group is the pivotal reference and affiliation group. Adolescents from these cultures have reservations regarding participation in a group outside of the extended family.

Possible stigmatization because of participation in groups may influence youngsters not to join groups in order to avoid a possible negative image of themselves. Adolescents interpret needing help as evidence of dependency, unworthiness, and vulnerability, which contradicts their desire to be independent and self-sustained. Immigrants perceive needing help as contradicting their fantasy of America as above all a country of freedom. Participation in a group is often seen by immigrant adolescents as an indication that they are not capable of coping with their own issues. This feeling may be intensified by reactions to classmates, friends, and school administration. For example, if members of an acculturation group from newcomers in a school are portrayed as "problematic," this image will stop adolescents who may have enjoyed the service from being associated with it.

In face of the aforementioned obstacles, the question arises of how to use the group work modality for working with adolescent immigrants in an effective way.

PRINCIPLES FOR EFFECTIVE GROUP WORK WITH ADOLESCENT IMMIGRANTS

Several principles proved to be helpful in planning and implementing group work services for adolescent immigrants.

First, it is important to provide services in community locations by offering groups in schools and in community centers. Many immigrants tend to be suspicious of mental health professionals affiliated with the establishment and are not as open as Westerners to the idea of therapy. Community-based groups help to diminish stigmatization and to normalize their use, thus making them accessible and attractive to a larger target population. Neutral locations also help gain parents' permission for their adolescent children to participate. Immigrant parents tend to approve educational, task-oriented group activities because of the high value their cultures of origin put on scholastic achievement. As many families were motivated to emigrate in order to provide their children with better prospects for the future, they tend to approve activities which they perceive to contribute to these prospects. School and school-related activities usually gain approval from immigrant parents, while expressing feelings in public and "just talking" are not.

Second, groups should be defined as "discussion groups" and focus on normal acculturation issues, even though over time some of them become more therapeutic in nature than others. Participants should be recruited both through reaching out directly in advertisements, by approaching natural groups, for example in lunchrooms and at Ping-Pong tables, and indirectly through guidance counselors and teachers of English as a second language. The facilitator can identify in the course of the group those individuals whose needs exceed the normative acceleration group process and required additional clinical interventions.

It is recommended that groups be offered in the native language of the participants. Homogenous groups were found to offer the optimum social context for rehabilitation immigrants' sense of identity (Halberstadt and Mandel, 1988, Mirsky and Prawer, 1992). Facilitating groups in the original language of group members serve two purposes. Many group members, especially newcomers, think in their native language for several years following immigration and struggle with finding correct words in English. This lack of fluency with the English language is a major stressor for immigrants (Zapf, 1991). Having a group in their language of origin facilitates the members' self-expression. It saves them from the double difficulty of discussing emotionally demanding issues in a foreign language with which they still do not feel comfortable and provides them with an opportunity to express their concerns and feelings more freely and easily. In addition, offering group services in their language of origin sends a positive message about the youngsters' culture of origin and validates the original cultural roots of group members as part of their current identity. Such a message promotes their self-esteem and is extremely important in helping the adolescent members perceive their original culture positively.

It is best for such groups to be facilitated by immigrant social workers from the same culture of origin as group members. Such workers have greater sensitivity to the teenagers' special needs since they know from personal experience what their clients are going through. The common experience prevents obstacles in communication which were described in refugee groups led by American workers (Glassman and Skolnik, 1984). Such group facilitators also serve as powerful role models because they represent the possibility "to make it" in the new culture.

Open-ended groups seem to work best for adolescent immigrants. Their flexibility allows the clients to manage their own attendance, thus reducing their anxiety about losing control over their lives and feeling the imposition of adults. The open-ended format also enables accommodation to the diverse needs of each adolescent.

RUSSIAN ADOLESCENTS PROJECT: AN ILLUSTRATION

The Russian Adolescents Project (RAP) of the Jewish Board of Families' and Children's' Services in Brighton Beach in New York City illustrates how the principles have been applied. In the past two decades the southern part of Brooklyn has absorbed two waves of immigrants from the former Soviet Union. Most of these are Jewish immigrants who came to the United States in two waves: the first in the late 1970s and the second in the early 1990s.

Currently, groups are meeting in public schools, parochial Jewish schools, and community centers. Groups meet during lunch periods, in after-school programs, in time slots designated for this purpose during the regular school schedule, or in evenings and on weekends.

The composition of groups may change in each meeting, even though, generally speaking, groups have a consistent core of participants. Group members often know each other and have intensive relationships outside of the group. Consequently, rules about confidentiality need to be repeated and emphasized constantly. Group facilitators are recent Russian immigrants who have a professional background in psychology, education, and related fields and are returning to school for the MSW degree. The program now includes twenty-six adolescent groups, five parents groups, and one teachers group.

Adolescent Groups

Ten to sixteen youngsters meet every week. Each meeting lasts from a half hour to an hour. Participants discuss issues of acculturation, identity, belonging, trust, and parent-adolescent relationships, all of which are universal to adolescents in general and are "amplified" in RAP by unique Russian features. For example, issues of trust toward adults that are typical of all adolescent groups are colored by their experience with the totalitarian and controlling Soviet regime; questions of intergender relationships are influenced by different Russian and American norms regarding relationship between men and women and acceptable sexual behavior; issues regarding conflicts with parents are heightened by their adapting to the liberal American norms faster than their parents, by their resentment toward parents who imposed emigration, and by their guilt feelings about their attitudes toward the parents.

Parents Groups

These groups provide mutual support and psychoeducation about raising adolescents in America. Participants learn about bicultural differences in norms, typical adolescent developmental processes in America, and appropriate disciplinary measures. Parents also support one another in their struggle to adapt to a new culture and to effectively parent their teenage children.

Teachers Group

Five teachers in the bilingual program meet and discuss students who have special problems as well as issues related to participating in a bilingual program. The idea of a bilingual program is highly debatable and produces intensive emotional reactions among supporters and opponents alike.

SUMMARY

Group work is an effective vehicle for providing services to immigrant adolescents. It offers them opportunities to address their cardinal issues at a time in their life when tensions pile up and resources for support shrink. Generally, to be effective a program should offer open-ended groups focused on normal issues in the participants' language of origin, facilitated by workers who themselves immigrated from the same culture in community-based, non-stigmatized environments. These guidelines need to be accommodated to fit the specific needs of all groups of immigrant adolescents, depending on the unique aspects of their cultures of origin and the levels of difference from the normal American culture. It is of utmost importance to evaluate the results of different programs with diverse groups of adolescent immigrants to further sharpen and develop our knowledge. With such knowledge we can tailor group work services to help this population deal with the doubly difficult challenges of adolescence and immigration.

REFERENCES

Baptiste, D. (1990). The treatment of adolescents and their families in cultural transition: Issues and recommendations. *Contemporary Family Therapy, 12* (1): 3-22.

Baptiste, D.A. (1993). Immigrant families, adolescents and acculturation: Insights for therapists. In B.H. Settles, D.E. Hanks, and M.B. Sussman (Eds.), *Families on the Move: Migration, Immigration, Emigration, and Mobility*. Binghamton, NY: The Haworth Press, Inc.

Berger, R. (1996). *From Comsomol to group work: Myths and realities in group work with immigrants from the former Soviet Union*. Paper presented at the Jewish Board of Families and Children Services, New York.

Blos, P. (1979). *The Adolescent Passage*. New York: International University Press.

Furnham, A. and Bochner, S. (1986). *Cultural Shock: Psychological Reactions to Unfamiliar Environments*. New York: Methuen.

Glassman, U. and Skolnik, L. (1984). The role of social group work in refugee resettlement. *Social Work with Groups, 7*(1): 45-62.

Gold, S.J. (1989). Differential adjustment among a new immigrant family members. *Journal of Contemporary Ethnography, 17*(4): 408-434.

Goldstein, E. (1979). Psychological adaptation of Soviet immigrants. *American Journal of Psychoanalysis, 39*(3): 257-263.

Goodenow, C. and Espin, O.M. (1993). Identity choices in immigrant adolescent females. *Adolescence, 28*(109): 173-184.

Grinberg, L. and Grinberg, I. (1989). *Psychoanalytic Perspectives on Migration and Exile*. New Haven, CT: Yale University Press.

Halberstadt, A. and Mandel, L. (1989). Group psychotherapy with Russia immigrants. In D. Halperin (Ed.), *Group Psychotherapy: New Paradigms and New Perspectives*. Chicago: Yearbook Medical Publishers.

Henry, S. (1992). *Group Skills in Social Work*. Pacific Grove, CA: Brooks.

Landau, J. (1983). Therapy with families in cultural transition. In M. McGoldrick, J.K. Pearce, and J. Giordano (Eds.), *Ethnicity and Family Therapy*. New York: Guilford.

Landau-Stanton, J. (1985). Adolescents, families, and cultural transition: A treatment model. In A. Mirkin and S. Koman (Eds.), *Handbook of Adolescents and Family Therapy*. New York: Gardner Press.

Leader, E. (1991). Why adolescent group therapy? *Journal of Child and Adolescent Group Psychotherapy, 1*(2): 81-93.

Lee, E. (1988). Cultural factors in working with Southeast Asian refugee adolescents. *Journal of Adolescence, 11*(2): 167-179.

Mirsky, J. and Prawer, L. (1992). *To Immigrate As an Adolescent.* Jerusalem: Van Leer Institute and Elka.

Shulman, L. (1993). *The Skills of Helping Individuals, Families, and Groups.* Itasca, IL: F.E. Peacock.

Zapf, K.M. (1991). Cross cultural transitions and wellness: Dealing with culture shock. *International Journal for the Advancement of Counselling, 14*(2): 105-119.

Chapter 11

Building Partnerships for Health Between Community Agencies and Schools: Two Communities, Two Cultures, Two Languages

Karen Culberg
Olga Medina
Rebecca Warner

INTRODUCTION

Early sexual activity and concomitant early pregnancy have received particular attention during the past few years as teen parents have become the target of much of the current welfare controversy. Immigrants have also received increased attention as a result of the emphasis to "end welfare as we know it." The needs of groups that have been scapegoated or ignored by mainstream society have been central to concerns of the Illinois Caucus for Adolescent Health (ICAH, formerly the Illinois Caucus on Teenage Pregnancy)[1] since its inception in 1977. ICAH is a membership organization working with grassroots organizations to highlight and develop culturally relevant and useful interventions that will provide models upon which administrative and legislative policy advocacy is built.

This chapter will describe the implementation of the parent component of a comprehensive sexuality curriculum in two schools, in two separate Chicago communities, one African American and one Mexican American. The story is one of adapting, refining, adding, and networking. Our approach is very much one that embraces the origins of social group work, for it requires that communities be assisted to find their own solutions. For the process to be meaningful when embarking upon a comprehensive sex education program, community members, including parents, must be involved at least in the early stages, and preferably throughout. Two of the staff of this project had worked together for four years at the time this project was implemented. A third staff member, although hired more recently, has spent many years as a certified family nurse practitioner, well grounded in community health needs and attitudes.

BACKGROUND OF PROJECT

Chicago is divided into seventy-seven community areas. These areas are used to report health statistics. The city has over 600 schools, none of which draw students exclusively from any one community area. Birth reports are given by community area. The size and complexity of the city require multiple systems and layers of management which ultimately reflect the highly bureaucratized nature of Chicago public schools. It is within this bureaucracy that the Illinois Caucus advocates for comprehensive health education including sexuality education. This requires both systemwide advocacy and local school involvement.

To bring any intervention into a school it is essential to have both the support of the principal and the endorsement of the parents. Parental support is gained in Chicago through endorsement by the Local School Council (LSC), a governing body elected every two years in each school and made up of elected teachers, community representatives, and parents. The LSC has the power to hire and fire the principal. This system was adopted with school reform in Chicago in 1989 and works variably. In schools where parents have a history of participation, understand the system, and are not intimidated by it, the LSC works very well. In schools where parents are new to Chicago, may have limited command of English, and are bewildered by the cultural conflicts between the old ways and the new, LSC may not function well. In very poor neighborhoods where parents have not been encouraged to be full participants in their own and their children's lives because of systemic problems (lack of employment opportunities, poor schools, generational poverty), the LSC also may not operate well. LSC approval must be gained to move ahead. Approval does not guarantee ongoing support, however, nor does initial enthusiasm by a principal.

The ICAH promotes comprehensive family life education within a healthy school which requires a realistic approach to the lives of young people and their families. Components of a healthy school are: a clean, safe school environment, nutritious food services, physical education, comprehensive health instruction, counseling and guidance services, staff health promotion, and parent, family and community involvement. (See Carnegie Council on Adolescent Development, 1989: Task Force on Education of Young Adolescents. *Turning Points: Preparing American Youth for the Twenty-First Century; The Report of the Task Force on Education of Young Adolescents.*)

This chapter is concerned primarily with family life education which is part of *health instruction.* The components of a healthy school are all interrelated, and the interventions we will describe depend primarily upon the last listed, namely *parent, family, and community involvement.* Community services are also integral, particularly health services and how to locate them in the community.

The ICAH received a grant from the Illinois Department of Public Health (IDPH) to pilot an "abstinence plus" curriculum. This grant was awarded after administrative advocacy by the ICAH that an "abstinence only" curriculum had received state funding without competitive bidding. Objections to this curriculum include concerns that it contains factual errors and it has a decidedly middle-class bias which will not resonate in the schools in areas of high poverty. For example, it suggests that young people entertain each other at dinner parties as a substitute for sexual experimentation. Further, the curriculum, with its insistence on abstinence, does not acknowledge that 42 percent of ninth graders who answered an Illinois Department of Public Health survey indicated that they were already sexually active. While that curriculum promotes "secondary virginity," there is little indication in the research that young people already engaging in sexual activity will cease. Rather, research does suggest that the provision of accurate information to already sexually active young people will result in more frequent contraceptive use.

In 1994 we selected the Oliver Wendell Holmes School in the Englewood community on the South side of Chicago to pilot the *Values and Choices* curriculum (Search Institute, n.d.). Englewood has one of the highest teen birth rates in Chicago, with 31.6 percent of the births in that community to teens. The social worker had worked in that school previously and knew the school nurse, parent-community representative, and former principal to be positive and anxious to provide comprehensive family life education. A new principal concerned about meeting state health education requirements was not obstructionist; however, because she was a new principal, she was not able to be as actively supportive as we had hoped.

We selected a SEICUS (Sex Education and Information Council of the United States) recommended curriculum, *Values and Choices* (V&C), produced by the Search Institute of Minneapolis (n.d.). V&C answered our criteria as it is comprehensive and abstinence-based with attention to contraception for information purposes. Further, it is values based and stresses seven basic values: equality, self-control, promise keeping, responsibility, respect, honesty, and social justice.

All lessons reinforce one or more of those values. This is a particularly appealing curriculum because it stresses equality between the sexes, which is essential in promoting and teaching the need for equality in dialogue between boys and girls concerning sexuality and related topics. Evaluation of this curriculum shows that those lessons retained for over three months include the belief in equality of the sexes and the information about sexually transmitted disease. Most sessions are taught with both sexes together which helps to normalize the atmosphere in which questions and concerns are raised. However, the student group was split into separate sessions for boys and girls for an opportunity to ask questions without embarrassment. Parent sessions are intended to be introduced concurrently with student units.

The curriculum was originally developed for seventh and eighth grade students. Because Holmes School comprises kindergarten through grade five, we consulted with the curriculum developers and were assured that modifications could be made to teach this to younger children. Modifications included elimination of the lessons on pregnancy and birth, and emphasis on those lessons dealing with values, with correct information and language, and designed to help young people talk to their parents and each other about this information.

Parents were invited to attend concurrent sessions to hear and approve—or disapprove—what their children would be learning. Very few parents have objected to this curriculum and those who do, object on religious grounds. Children whose parents do not wish for them to participate are able to go to another classroom.

The parent sessions are ideally targeted to parents of children receiving the curriculum. At Holmes School all parents who happened to be in the building—and there are many who are paid by Chapter 1 funds—were encouraged to attend. We supplied refreshments and prizes as incentives. Our participation rate was high even though many of the parents did not have children in the fourth or fifth grade classes. We justified this because this is a close-knit community, with many kinship ties. Children have siblings or cousins who would be learning the curriculum and we reasoned that an educational function would be served through broad parent participation. In addition, some parents are working and some families are dysfunctional, both working against parent participation.

Sessions taught to the students were conducted by a (female) family nurse practitioner and a (male) graduate student. Parent sessions were taught by the social worker or the social worker and nurse or another health educator in combination. Due to constraints of time we condensed the fifteen lessons into five sessions for both children and parents. This number of sessions is less than optimal for children but included more parent sessions than the Search Institute had provided in its own trainings.

Sessions were scheduled to last for one hour. Our format included a brief presentation of information followed by an interactive session with parents in which they could express their feelings about content, gain factual information and express concerns about what had just been presented. Parents in both schools were uniformly concerned that their children should have as much information as possible. In all of the sessions at Holmes School the sessions were lively and well attended.

What was the result? Parents told us that they were better able to talk to their children and to each other about sensitive issues. They welcomed handouts to take home and discuss with their children and with each other. One mother told us that she and her husband were both uncomfortable talking to their child when she brought home "nasty" pictures. The school nurse asked us to talk to the parents about how to respond to their own discomfort. We did, and the next week the mother who had been embarrassed to talk to her child reported that she had a conversation with her child about the body parts which had previously embarrassed her. Another mother was quite upset that this material was being introduced at the fifth grade level. Her daughter, she said, is of the age when she should be focused on what she will be when she grows up and not "this stuff." The school nurse, who sat in at all sessions, explained the strategy behind drug prevention education and sex education to the parents: risky behaviors are best discussed before they are likely to occur, when communication is possible and we might eliminate or postpone those behaviors. Many teachable moments resulted from the interaction between parents, outside staff, school nurse, and invited community agencies.

Along with seventy-seven distinct community areas, Chicago is a city of neighborhoods, and as such is highly stratified by race and ethnicity. The population of Englewood is 99 percent African American, and the population of Holmes School is 100 percent African American. By contrast, South Lawndale, also known as Little Village, is 85 percent Latino, with most of the residents having come from Mexico. Twenty-Sixth Street, as it runs through Little Village, could be in Mexico if the buildings were not vintage Chicago brick. Madero School is two blocks north of Twenty-Sixth Street and the population is reflective of the neighborhood. The ICAH was invited to come to the school during the summer of 1994 by the principal to discuss her concerns regarding early sexual activity and need for information by the children at Madero School. This school is composed of grades five through eight in a former high school building which has been converted to accept overflow students from McCormick School, some blocks away. This is significant because until recently the school was called McCormick Branch, and as such parents did not feel they received their due, but were primarily a stepchild of the other school.

To review our lesson from Holmes: it is mandatory that both the principal and LSC be supportive of any new endeavor. We felt very confident that Madero would be a receptive school because the principal had invited us and assured us that parents were anxious for information for their children. The principal asked the school community representative to arrange a meeting for us with parents. During the same summer we returned to the school to meet parents and begin to perform a needs assessment. Our agenda changed when we entered the school and saw that those mothers who had come had brought their adolescent daughters. The mothers wanted their daughters to have information quickly, and in their presence, if possible.

We asked the mothers, "What do you worry about most for your children?" To the students we asked, "What do you worry about most for your friends?" The mothers replied that they were concerned about changing relationships between parents and children—their children seem to be losing respect for parents; that they will not finish school; who they choose as friends. The daughters answered that it worries them when their friends are in gangs; pregnancy and drugs; about schoolwork.

We asked them to respond to a list of potential discussion items. Both mothers and daughters answered that communications in the family were the greatest concern. The mothers answered in equal numbers that talking about sex with their children was of concern, whereas only half of the daughters were interested in talking about sex. Later, however, during discussion both mothers and daughters said it would be better for the young women to meet alone to have their questions answered. Sexual abuse and relations between mother and child ranked next with the same amount of concern.

We asked what resources for health and safety should be included in a neighborhood. Mothers replied: places where our kids can be active, some training for young girls in home economics, communication in general and with neighbors, and cleaning. Students, while reiterating that there shouldn't be gangs also said, "more friendly people," and "people who care." In the course of our time at Madero School we learned that parents must come a distance to the school since it is far from their neighborhood school. Many do not want to travel so far. For those who speak only Spanish it is uncomfortable to go outside of their immediate neighborhood. Even more important, we learned that many of them come to the school to pick up their children at the end of the day because the distance between their homes and the school means that children have to cross rival gang territory. Going back and forth to the school once a day is enough.

Madero parent sessions were conducted in Spanish; however, the language in the video accompanying *Values and Choices* is English. It is not the same to hear about information which is taboo in the old culture discussed in a language which is not your own. The Caucus has proposed to the Search Institute that funding be sought to develop the video in Spanish which will remove one source of distance from the process. The parents who participated in the sessions obviously enjoyed them, but we never had the numbers at Madero School because of the factors mentioned. We also learned that even when the principal overtly supports the notion, if he or she is not able to remove impediments that exist in the community, a full-blown effort will not get off the ground. At Madero, as at Holmes, the nurse practitioner and graduate student taught five sixth grade classes. In contrast to the children at Holmes School the children at Madero School were very shy in asking questions. An envelope that was made available for anonymous questions was always full at Holmes School. At Madero School during eight forty-minute presentations to 130 sixth graders, only fifteen written questions were submitted. When we began meeting with the parents in session we showed them the questions their children had asked. Their response was similar to the Holmes' parents: if our children have these questions and are thinking about these things, they should have a place to learn correct information.

To review: we learned that to have a true community-based effort, planning should include all players. Even though the entire school community shared the same concerns as the principal at Madero, problems of travel, distance, and safety rendered possible solutions to some of the problems unlikely. Parents asked Caucus staff if the session could be held at McCormick School, and even though there appear to be many political issues between the two schools, it appears that to provide parents with information, it must be provided at the site closest to home. Our lessons inform our advocacy.

DEVELOPMENT OF CURRENT INTERVENTION

Our work with parents in the program contributed to the establishment of a truly comprehensive, community-driven effort in another Chicago Latino community. This project, *Proyecto Intercambio,* brings interventions developed and evaluated in Mexico to two Chicago Spanish-speaking communities. Our belief is that materials developed in Spanish, and delivered in that language to individuals whose first language is Spanish, will be more acceptable to new residents in recent immigrant communities. This is even more important at a time when punishing legislation is directed toward many immigrants, including those who came to this country intending to live as full participants.

NOTE

1. The name was changed in 1993 to reflect a broader emphasis on health. While adolescent pregnancy and parenting remain central to the mission of the organization, the shift allows us to consider young men and holistic health issues, of which reproductive health is but one.

REFERENCES

Carnegie Council on Adolescent Development. Task Force on Education of Young Adolescents (1989). *Turning Points: Preparing American Youth for the Twenty-First Century: The Report of the Task Force on Education of Young Adolescents.* Washington, DC: Author.
Search Institute (n.d.). *Value and Choices Curriculum.* Minneapolis: Author.
Sex Education and Information Council of the United States. New York.

Chapter 12

Multiple Intelligences
in Group Work Activities:
Reaffirming Our Roots

Kendra J. Garrett
Barbara E. Berger

Many individuals with good verbal skills benefit greatly from the traditional therapeutic methods of talking about problems. Others have strengths in different areas. Recent research indicates that, in addition to verbal intelligence, there are actually six other ways in which people learn and grow. In other words, there are multiple intelligences (Gardner, 1983). Group workers have rarely relied on discussion alone, often using program activities to help clients grow and change. The purpose of this chapter is to review our history of using program activities in groups and to explore the connection between such activities and the way people learn.

Exercises and activities in group work can serve many purposes. Activities can facilitate verbal communication, reduce stress, satisfy the need for creativity, stimulate problem solving, enhance the development of relationships, improve social skills, enhance self-esteem, and allow leaders to assess the needs of members in the group (Northen, 1988). Activities also encourage human contact, help members rehearse tasks, increase tolerance of differences, and introduce difficult topics (Shulman, 1971). They are also helpful in working with groups whose members are action-prone, such as children and adolescents. In those groups, having something to do reduces anxiety about sharing personal information and being accepted by others (Northen, 1988). Activities are particularly helpful with members who have challenges to verbal communication such as speech delays, language barriers, or shyness. Malekoff (1988) describes the use of goal-directed activities to problem solve and to gain interpersonal skills in a group of preadolescent children who had difficulty using discussion.

The use of activities or "program" with groups has a rich, albeit fragmented, history. The use of program activities began in settlement houses and national service organizations (Coyle, 1948) where workers used recreational games to teach, socialize, and play with children. The use of activities continues today, although we now are more likely to call them simulations, games, activities, tasks, and role-plays instead of "program" (Middleman, 1979). Gisela Konopka (1963) pointed out that group work and recreating were mistakenly considered interchangeable for many years. For a time social workers needed to find a higher purpose or rationale for their activities so it didn't appear to be just "fun and games." Yet some of the negative reactions to the use of activities in group work, according to Shulman (1971), come in reaction to exaggerated claims of growth through their use. Shulman suggested that the *most* important issue related to activities is individualizing them to complement and enhance clients' learning and expression. Discerning what activities are available to group members and why has continued to be an important question, and the answer has become more complex and varied as knowledge of group theory and respect for diversity increases.

As group work changed over time from a focus on participation in a democracy and social change to a focus on individual problems, workers began to use discussion more and activities less. Groups became more worker-directed and made less frequent use of members' preference and interests (Middleman, 1979). Yet, program has never truly left social work groups. Middleman pointed out that in 1979 we were just beginning to appreciate the intuitive, deductive, and dialectic patterns of thinking. Eastern modes of knowing were no longer seen as inferior to the ways of science. These broadened ways of thinking and learning expanded our repertoire of activities and our rationale for using them. All of these new "insights" seem to be resurfacing in the discussion of "multiple intelligences."

MULTIPLE INTELLIGENCES

It is our assumption that, at least at some level, education is a component of all treatment groups, whether they be self-help, education, support, or therapeutic. Most educational activities used in schools fall into one of two traditional categories: verbal/linguistic or logical/mathematical (Gardner, 1993). Verbal/linguistic activities involve the use of oral or written language. Examples include reading, writing, and discussion. Mathematical/logical activities use numbers and reasoning skills to determine patterns of relationships, predict outcomes and consequences, generalize, and test hypotheses. Examples include experimenting, problem solving, and outlining (Larseth and Tebben, 1995). However, increasing evidence indicates that these two approaches to education address only a small portion of an individual's total intelligence. Gardner (1983, 1993) in his work on multiple intelligences has identified five additional kinds of intelligence. These are:

- *Visual/spatial.* The ability to visualize, represent, and locate people and objects within three-dimensional space (as in art).
- *Body/kinesthetic.* The use of balance, coordination, strength, and agility to express ideas or emotions (as in dance).
- *Musical/rhythmical.* Use of musical forms and patterns as forms of expression (as in music or drumming).
- *Interpersonal.* Understanding distinctions among others and noticing nonverbal communication of moods, temperaments, motivations, and intentions so as to interact effectively with others (as in empathizing or mediating).
- *Intrapersonal.* Identifying and labeling one's own emotions and understanding how they guide behavior (as in creative thought or dreaming).

As a result of his research in teaching children through the use of multiple intelligences, Gardner (1993) has identified five ways to present content so as to tap into the several intelligences.

1. In a *narrative* approach, one uses storytelling or poetry.
2. When using a *logical-quantitative* approach, a teacher introduces logic, mathematical concepts, deductive reasoning and scientific methods.

3. The *foundation* approach emphasizes a philosophical understanding in which basic questions are discovered about the nature of a subject.
4. The *esthetic* approach uses spatial knowledge, artistic expression, and music.
5. An *experiential* approach emphasizes kinesthetic "doing" in which students participate in and explore the topic.

The use of multiple intelligences is a holistic way of viewing learners. Instead of focusing on verbal/linguistic and mathematical/logical presentation of subjects to be learned, teachers use a variety of approaches which allow students to participate in a subject, perhaps by attending a museum (experiential approach), or through a foundational approach, in which the student works to uncover questions about the nature of a subject. Teaching is often done through the use of projects in which students pursue subjects of interest by creating, organizing, and exploring material and presenting a final product to others. Students also develop process folios (similar to portfolios) which include not only finished work, but also the partial products and false starts that helped them learn about their topics. Because people in real life often work collaboratively to solve problems, students often work together to find answers, thus building on strengths of group members (Gardner, 1993).

Assessment techniques for the various intelligences are under investigation. A profile system, in which the relative strengths of the seven intelligences are listed, is one possibility. This assessment would include a discussion of the student's skills in each area and some suggestions for making improvements. These areas would be assessed in the context of everyday activities, particularly those which have relevance to adulthood and problem solving. Intelligences would not be assessed through the use of paper and pencil standardized tests (Gardner, 1993).

GROUP WORK AND MULTIPLE INTELLIGENCES

Many clients come to social workers because of difficulty with two of Gardner's seven intelligences: inter- and intrapersonal. Interpersonal intelligence, as stated earlier, is the ability to notice differences among others' moods, temperaments, motivations, and intentions and to use this information in relating to others. Interpersonal intelligence can be directly expressed in personal interaction and does not rely on other intelligences to be expressed. An example of an interpersonal activity that promotes empathy and effective interaction with others is "Role Taking," a small group activity in which the facilitator helps group members identify a conflict situation from their own lives and asks two members to act it out. After a minute or two, members switch sides and symbolically move into the chair formerly occupied by the other person. They continue the role-play, now taking on the role of the other participant.

Intrapersonal intelligence is the ability to discriminate among and to level one's own emotions and to understand how they guide behavior. Intrapersonal intelligence cannot be readily observed and relies on some other form of intelligence, such as music, linguistic ability, or art, in order to be communicated (Gardner, 1993). It is the premise of multiple intelligences theory that strengths in one or more intelligences can be used to teach and help people grow. Perhaps the other five intelligences can best be used in helping people grow in inter- and intrapersonal areas.

FIVE ENTRY POINTS TO IMPROVED INTER- AND INTRAPERSONAL SKILLS

Interpersonal Skills

In helping members improve in interpersonal areas, group facilitators might use the five learning approaches identified by Gardner to identify activities and projects to help each member grow to meet his or her goals. A *narrational* approach might include asking members to tell or write a story about a friendship or write a poem about getting along with others or about loneliness. The activity "Feeling Wall" promotes participants' designation and expression of feelings and emotions that helps them make connections between feelings and behaviors. It is suitable for an entire group. Large, long sheets of brown or white wrapping paper and various writing materials (markers, crayons, pencils, etc.) are needed. In step one the facilitator tapes large sheets of paper together to form a large writing surface. These are taped to the wall at participant's eye level. The facilitator explains to participants that they can use this "Feeling Wall" and the available materials to express themselves in words or pictures. In step two (more appropriate with teen or adult participants), the participants volunteer to make connections between their feelings and behavior (Adapted from Watkins and Durant, 1996).

The worker could also include *mathematical/logical* activities such as logical deductions about getting along or creating in-depth relationships. Members make deductions regarding others' feelings from observing pictures. Members also develop logical hypotheses as to what actions might be appropriate in certain circumstances relating to the feelings or needs of others. An example is the activity "Individual Decision Making with Group Input." The goal is to promote participants' ability to think logically about a problem, potential solutions, and consequences of solution options as well as consequences of inaction. This activity is suitable for six to eight participants. Chalkboard or flip chart, and chalk or markers are needed. A group member asks for the group's attention to a decision-making dilemma he or she is facing. On the board or flip chart, the participant, with assistance from the group, lists the alternate decision possibilities, implications, and consequences of each option as well as exploration of inaction. The participant takes the information generated by the discussion under advisement and reports back to the group what decision has been made, if and when it occurs.

From a *foundational* entry point, group members could consider what friendship is and of what it consists, asking philosophical questions about the nature of interpersonal relationships. Using an *esthetic* approach, group members could write music or create artwork relating to their ideas of getting along and forming relationships. The activity "Rap a Feeling" illustrates music and song as a way to address relationships. The worker prepares cards, each displaying a feeling word. The group is divided into subgroups of four or six. Each group picks a "feeling card." The group creates a rap song depicting that feeling. Each group works for ten minutes then presents its rap to the entire group. An *experiential* approach would involve simply doing activities with others (e.g., playing basketball or bowling) as a way of building relationships.

Intrapersonal Skills

Addressing intrapersonal issues could use a similar framework. A *narrational* approach would include writing poetry about one's thoughts and feelings or telling a story about personal experiences. A *kinesthetic* approach might be the "Strike a Pose" activity. The goal is to illustrate metaphorically by two poses, the movement associated with change and specifically with movement and posture that is associated with greater freedom and flexibility. One or more instant cameras and film are needed. Participants form pairs, using instant cameras to take two photographs of each other. One pose depicts, "As I was," or "As I am," one depicts, "As I would like to be." (The poses are often overstated.) After the snapshots are completed the partners discuss their significance with one another. Then the pairs reunite with the other pairs and each individual shares his or her poses and their meaning with the group (An adaptation of a Visual Transitions activity in Wadeson, Durkin, and Perach, 1989).

A *mathematical/logical* approach would include a logical discussion about the benefits of self-knowledge or creating hypotheses (and testing them out) about how people grow in personal insight. *Foundational* approaches might include discussions about the nature of knowing oneself or the state and purpose of understanding emotions. Group members could express their thoughts and feelings about themselves nonverbally through sculpting, music, or an *esthetic* approach. *Experience* might include meditation or self-reflection. The activity "Goal Attainment Barriers: A Pictorial Representation" promotes participants' awareness of obstacles that prevent them from attaining goals. This activity is suitable for an entire group. Materials needed are large and small pieces of paper, and crayons, markers, or paint. Individuals are instructed to select paper and materials and depict a barrier that they believe stands in the way of realization of an important life goal. Then participants "pair off" with another group member and discuss their work, or discuss it with the entire group (An adaptation of an art therapy exercise for depressed women in Wadeson, Durkin, and Perach, 1989).

Such approaches are not new to group workers. For example, the use of cognitive therapy to treat depression can be considered a way of using verbal/linguistic skills (such as self-talk) and mathematical/logical skills (such as examining one's hypotheses about oneself) to change patterns of thinking. And social workers have often used music, dance, and art to help people express emotions. What is, perhaps, new is the systematic thinking about applying *seven* intelligences and five learning approaches to create program activities in treatment groups.

SEVEN INTELLIGENCES AND PROGRAM ACTIVITIES

Of course, social workers do not limit their group work to just treatment groups. For example, personal growth, self-help, and socialization groups could use multiple intelligences and learning approaches to help determine a wide range of activities so as to give group members many different opportunities. One of the authors participated in a woman's spiritual growth group that used storytelling and discussion (verbal/linguistic); problem solving and symbolism (mathematical/logical); sculpting and drawing (visual/spatial); dance and drama (body/kinesthetic); chanting and drumming (musical/rhythmical); empathizing and relating (interpersonal); and mediation and reflection (intrapersonal). This group was able to use all seven kinds of intelligence in helping the members grow.

By considering the prominent intelligences of group members in the beginning of a group, leaders can become aware of the ways group members learn. Many activities tap into several intelligences at once. Such activities may be used in groups whose members have different areas of intellectual strength. In groups in which members have a predominant intelligence style, the worker should be aware of minority styles and design additional activities to target members who do not share the dominant learning patterns. It is important to vary activities so as to tap into various members' learning strengths and help them use these strengths to grow.

Of course the use of purposeful activities in group work is not new. But Gardner (1983, 1993) has provided us with an additional way of considering which activities are best suited to different group members and a framework for developing group activities that tap into the various intelligences. Activities have long been used in group work, however, and appear to be as popular among group workers as ever. Perhaps the use of the framework of learning approaches can help us be more systematic in choosing activities which will tap into members' strengths.

REFERENCES

Coyle, G. (1948). *Group Work with American Youth.* New York: Harper.

Gardner, H. (1983). *Frames of Mind: The Theory of Multiple Intelligences.* New York: Basic Books.

Gardner H. (1993). *Multiple Intelligence: The Theory in Practice.* New York: Basic Books.

Konopka, G. (1963). *Social Group Work: A Helping Process.* Englewood Cliffs, NJ: Prentice Hall.

Larseth, D. and Tebben, S. (1995, February). Engaging the multiple mind through assessment. Paper presented at the Bush Regional Collaboration in Faculty Development, Minneapolis, MN.

Malekoff, A. (1988). The preadolescent prerogative: Creative blends of discussion and activity in group treatment. *Social Work with Groups, 10*(4), 61-81.

Middleman, R. (1979). The use of program: Review an update. *Social Work with Groups, 3*(3), 5-23.

Northen, H. (1988). *Social Work with Groups.* New York: Columbia University Press.

Shulman, L. (1971). "Program" in group work: Another look. In W. Schwartz and S. Zalba (Eds.), *The Practice of Group Work.* New York: Columbia University Press, 221-240.

Wadeson, H., Durkin, J., and Perach, D. (1989). *Advances in Art Therapy.* New York: John Wiley and Sons.

Watkins, K. and Durant, L. (1996). *Working with Children and Families Affected by Substance Abuse.* New York: The Center for Applied Research in Education.

Chapter 13

Circles: Intergroup Bridging Using the Dynamic Circles Exercise (DCE)

Lea Kacen

The Dynamic Circles Exercise (DCE) is an elaboration on the Fishbowl technique, based on theoretical principles from existentialist theory, Gestalt theory, and learning theory. Four examples of the DCE applications are presented: a case involving drug addicts and third year social work students; a case adding new volunteers to a group of veteran volunteers, confronting mothers and fathers of handicapped children in couple group intervention; and settling a conflict within an interdisciplinary team of workers. The strengths and dangers of the DCE, as well as the nature of the exercise are discussed. The need for intergroup bridging may be apparent in situations involving integration of immigrants from different countries and cultures. Bridging is also needed in other situations of intergroup conflict, for example: tension between two rival street gangs, work in multidisciplinary teams, and various therapy situations, such as social integration of reformed drug addicts, criminals, and victim-offender mediation (Mika, 1995; Bargal and Bar, 1992, 1994).

This chapter is a modified and combined version of two papers originally published in *Simulation & Gaming: An International Journal of Theory, Practice, and Research 29*(1), pp. 88-100, and 101-104, 1998. Published by permission of the editor of *S&G*.

The author would like to thank Ela Melamed, Michal Ben-Kochav, Roni Eyal, and all the students who took part in her Group Leadership Skills Seminar, and who helped in developing the exercise by practicing it in the class and in the field. She also wishes to thank Gita Sofer and the *Simulation and Gaming* reviewers for their useful comments.

Being involved in intergroup bridging attempts means taking risks and being ready to act without being certain of the process's results. Mistakes in the bridging process could cause an escalation of tension and endanger the very existence of both groups.

In fact, it is possible to position results of attempts at intergroup bridging on a continuous line, which would be anchored at one end by "peaceful coexistence," i.e., two groups existing side by side, each with mutual respect for the individuality of the other (Thalhofer, 1993), and at the other end by "animosity," i.e., the groups becoming intransigent and introverted to the extent of alienating themselves from their surroundings (Chang, 1992).

To reduce the "price of mistakes" (Crookall, Oxford, and Saunders, 1987) in unsuccessful rapprochement attempts, the exercise allows the groups to learn the significance of bridging for themselves, within a protected environment. This chapter presents the exercise's theoretical basis, principles, and applications. Real world examples are described.

INTERGROUP CONFLICT

The ways in which groups relate to each other influence members' behavior, as well as the behavior and attitudes of the group's surrounding (Johnson and Johnson, 1991; Tajfel, 1982). The more an intergroup relationship is measured according to win-lose criteria, the greater the effect on the behavior of the individual group members (Sherif, 1966). Competitive relationships can create intergroup conflicts that express themselves by emphasizing the difference and distance between the groups, by stereotyping members of the other group, and by making generalizations with regard to everything concerned with it, all of which can produce ideal "scapegoat" conditions (Johnson and Johnson, 1991).

Lewin (1953) claims that behavioral changes resulting from intergroup conflicts demand conceptual changes within the group itself and, primarily, changes in the self-perception of each group member. Thus, for example, society depicts a stereotypical image of drug addicts as losers, people who are not worth wasting time on (Rugel, 1991). This type of concept prevents society from accepting rehabilitated drug addicts and may deny them the chance of becoming equal members of society. In this case, bridging between rehabilitated drug addicts and "normal" society can take place only when members of both groups succeed in changing individual self-perceptions. Changes in one's self-perception can best take place within a supportive environment that permits such a process. The exercise described here offers these conditions.

THE DYNAMIC CIRCLES EXERCISE (DCE)

The DCE is based on the three basic steps of the Fishbowl technique; however, a dynamic component is added. At the beginning of the exercise, members of one group sit in an inner circle and members of the other groups sit in an outer circle. The inner circle begins a discussion of issues concerning their stances and feelings toward the process of rapprochement to the other group, in ways appropriate to them (the inner circle), while the outer circle observes and listens (see Figure 13.1a). The observers are allowed to ask questions of the working group and the latter may decide whether to relate to any point raised in the questions or to ignore them. In any case, at this stage any direct dialogue between the members of both groups or between individuals belonging to the separate groups is categorically forbidden. In step #2, the groups change places and tasks (see Figure 13.1b).

Unlike the Fishbowl technique, group members are allowed to move freely from one circle to another during steps #1 and #2, to investigate or to express their attitudes toward the other group (see Figure 13.1d). In other words, all changes in members' attitudes toward the other group must be given physical expression through the seating arrangements. The goal is to illustrate these changes both physically and visually.

In step #3, both groups sit in a single large circle for debriefing (see Figure 13.1c). After each participant has had his or her turn, an open discussion may take place with the aim of connecting what happened during the meeting to the everyday reality of each group member.

Steps #1 and #2 are meant to emphasize the differences and similarities as well as the dynamic characteristic of the situation. These differences and similarities, together with their effect on

FIGURE 13.1. The Dynamic Circles Exercise

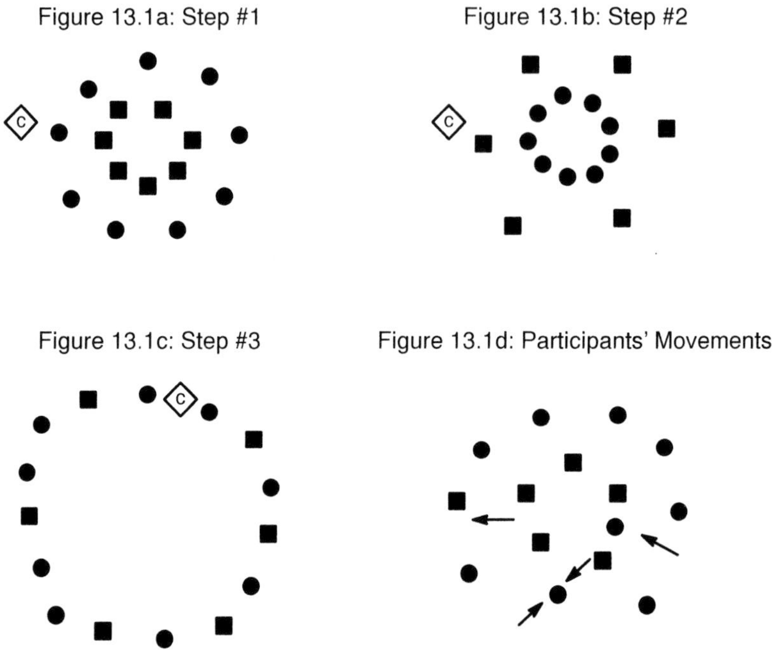

Figure 13.1a: Step #1

Figure 13.1b: Step #2

Figure 13.1c: Step #3

Figure 13.1d: Participants' Movements

reality, are discussed in step #3, and ways are examined through which it might be possible to create bridges between the two groups, both in the "here and now" of the training program and in the actual reality.

Rules of the Exercise

The rules of the DCE differentiate it from the Fishbowl technique. These rules define the dynamic component that is created between the circles when the aim is to turn them into a single large circle. The following rules must be observed, to create a protected environment in which one group of people is able to cope with the experience of being bridged to another group.

1. A personal agreement, regarding this exercise, must be drawn with each of the groups' participants. When the entire training is

designed with this exercise the agreement must be made as part of the group construction.

2. The exercise must be explained in advance, using appropriate practice.

3. At the beginning of the exercise, participants are obliged to sit in two separate circles—this signifies their singularity.

4. During steps #1 and #2 the group's members are allowed to move freely from one circle to another and between them, to investigate or to express their attitudes toward the other group. The aim of these moves is to illustrate these changes both physically and visually.

5. Each group is allotted a specific length of time for work in the inner circle. A time period of ten to fifteen minutes is preferable; this prevents the outer circle from becoming bored.

6. Those people sitting in the outer circle and observing the activity in the inner circle are not permitted to directly respond to what is being said. They are, however, allowed to ask questions. Members of the inner circle are allowed to either relate to the questions or to ignore them.

7. Direct dialogue between the two groups must not be permitted during steps #1 and #2. This is to allow the inner group a distinct time period to examine its positions, and the outer group the possibility to listen only. Direct dialogue is liable to draw the groups into positions of defense or power conflicts, thus distancing them further from the ultimate aim of the exercise.

8. In the debriefing stage (step #3), both groups sit in a single large circle. In order for the discussion to focus on the "here and now," the participants must begin their discourse with the sentence: "When I was in the outer circle, I felt . . ." or "When I was in the inner circle, I felt . . ." After each participant has had his or her turn, an open discussion may take place with the aim of connecting what happened during the meeting to the everyday reality of each group member.

9. The coordinator does not join the circles, except during the third phase. This will preserve the neutrality necessary to achieve the confidence of both groups, to allow him or her to ensure that the rules of the exercise are observed, and to help each of the groups in its work.

10. The groups are allowed to decide on new rules during the work process.

The Role of the Coordinator

The coordinator determines the exercise's basic rules and draws up suitable, separate, individual contracts with each of the participants and with the two groups with each other. He or she ensures the rules of the exercise and helps the groups to work when they are in the center and in the large circle. It is recommended that the coordinator help the members of the inner circle to focus on themselves, their thoughts and feelings, and avoid a discussion of those who sit in the outer circle. It is the coordinator's task to protect members of the group from possible dangers. To achieve the goals of the exercise, it is imperative that the coordinator preserve a maximum level of neutrality throughout the exercise.

Symbolizing Intergroup Bridging Through the DCE

The term "to bridge" is used here to stress the dynamic characteristic of the exercise that is aimed at building a bridge between groups. This bridge gives group members the opportunity to cross to the other side without the necessity of removing obstacles that lie in the way. In this way, participants can move freely between the circles, examining their own feelings, while at the same time examining the other circle's willingness to accept them.

During this process, intergroup bridging will express itself in obvious changes in the seating arrangements. Members of the various circles will move their chairs in such a way that the level of physical proximity between them and the other circle expresses the level of social/emotional closeness they feel for the other group at that particular time. Maximum openness and acceptance are expressed by taking the chair and physically joining the other group. Making this move means that they are willing to accept the other group's behavioral norms.

Each physical move that takes place between the two circles and within them serves to signify some kind of process in the relationship between the two groups and will be used as a basis for discussion.

Theoretical Background

DCE is based on principles firmly lodged in several theories. The first is the existentialist principle of the "here and now." By allowing members to bring life experiences into the "here and now" of the group, it is easier to direct the intervention toward constant expansion of self-awareness. This principle demands that, on the one hand, the participants take responsibility for their actions in the present while, on the other hand, does not allow them to retain explanations from their past (Rubinstein, 1990).

The second is the Gestalt principle of emphasizing the differences. According to this principle, emphasizing the differences and boundaries may contribute to a harmonious interaction later on. Emphasizing the disparities and contrasts between various behavior pattern components clears up antagonistic situations, reduces anxieties, and creates the desire to come together, based on acceptance and cooperation (Serok, 1980; Lewin, 1989).

The third is the modeling principle, which is borrowed from learning theory. According to this theory, exposing one person to another whether really, symbolically, or imaginatively, helps the person learn new behavior patterns and skills, while reducing the anxiety connected with the object, the group, or the place (Towle, 1954; Yalom, 1985).

The last is the inductive learning principle. Inductive learning from one's own experience is most effective, since learners discover for themselves what they have to learn through the existential experience (Pfieffer and Jones, 1975).

Examples

DCE has been used by the researcher, her students, and colleagues in a large number of groups and situations. Although no empirical study has yet been done of the efficacy of DCE in intergroup bridging, it should be pointed out that changes in group members' attitudes toward others have been observed and some conflicts and strains were resolved in all the cases. Moreover, it was learned that it is possible to use DCE for a number of objectives:

1. Personal changes
2. Merging two groups into one

3. Introducing concerns of two groups to each other and
4. Settling conflicts.

The aims of DCE determine its inclusion as part of the program. It is possible to include it for the entire duration of the intervention program, or for a few meetings only, or only once under certain circumstances. The following are a number of examples demonstrating the uses of DCE for different objectives and for different lengths of time.

Example #1: Victims of Drug Abuse
and Students of Social Work:
An Example of Personal Change

In 1990, a group of three students used the Dynamic Circle Exercise with a group of drug addicts undergoing a rehabilitation process. One group consisted of nine adult male drug addicts, undergoing a rehabilitation process under the supervision of the Beer-Sheva Adult Probation Services. Their ages ranged between twenty-two and thirty-seven; some were married, some were not. The other group consisted of three female third-year students of social work, doing their fieldwork with the Adult Probation Services. The groups held a total of eight meetings, the first of which was devoted to getting familiarized with each other, and explaining the "rules of the exercise." All the others were planned according to the DCE principle. The groups worked without the help of a coordinator, although the students received counseling.

During the first meetings, the drug addicts, sitting in the inner circle, discussed their world, their daily confrontation with their drug addiction, and their previous way of life. There was an obvious refraining from discussing the present. The group of students, on the other hand, pointed out their professional status and their relationship with the other group as result of this status. At this point, the distance between the two groups was most obvious.

The differences between these two worlds peaked during the third meeting, when one of the addicts sitting in the outer circle asked the students in the inner circle: "What would you do if one of you had a brother who was a drug addict?" One of the students replied, quite spontaneously: "Heaven forbid!" This answer pointed to the reality of "here and now" differences and the huge void between the two groups. Moreover, it exposed for the first time the student's human aspect of having stances and feelings in regard to drug addicts. The veil of professionalism was lifted and the way was paved for a more evenly matched, humane encounter.

During the discussion in step #3, a possible channel for bridging between the two groups was identified. This change signified the first stage in the life of the group, and made possible more profound relationships in the ensuing meetings. "The subjective component of a meeting between two worlds is shown to be of central importance in the process," wrote the students in their report to their counselor. "Not only did we look at each other, but from this stage onward, we were better able to feel and sense the world of the drug addict. This process consisted of emotional involvement which did not threaten our professional senses."

Success was partial. At the end of the process, one of the addicts entered the students' circle, where he was accepted as a member. Another addict joined a rehabilitation program, after nineteen years of addiction. Another went to prison, and yet another went back on drugs. The others dropped out at various stages of the group process.

Example #2: Integrating New Volunteers
into a Group of Veteran Volunteers:
An Example of Using DCE to Unite Two Groups

The Ministry of Defense Rehabilitation Units in Israel are volunteers to help widows and bereaved families come to terms with the day-to-day problems of their bereavement. These volunteers receive guidance and support within the framework of small groups. Two such groups operated in the southern region of the country.

It became necessary to include new volunteers in the two groups, who had been working as closed groups for a period of six years. The problem was how to integrate the new volunteers into the groups of veterans in the shortest possible time and with maximum efficiency, taking into consideration the differences in ages and experience between the two groups. We used the DCE to speed up the process. From the very beginning, working in circle bared all the differences between the two groups, defined the boundaries, and made it possible to identify possible channels for bridging, such as ways for transferring knowledge from the veteran group to the new group, pairing off house calls—when the pair consists of one veteran volunteer and one new volunteer, etc.

In the other group, the one in which integration of the new volunteers was not done in this way—the coordinators encountered resistance on the side of the veteran volunteers, who felt the continued existence of their primary group was threatened. There was even a fear at one stage that the veteran volunteers would drop out of the group.

Example #3: Using DCE for Introducing the Concerns
of Two Groups to Each Other: Fathers and Mothers
of Handicapped Children

Eight couples (four men and four women) took part in the parents' group. The group's aim was to provide strength and support in coping with a severely handicapped child (severely handicapped: a child suffering from a number of handicaps—badly developmentally disabled, hyperactive, physical disabilities, deafness, and autism). DCE was used at the beginning of group activity, with the fathers constituting one circle, and the mothers making up the other. Differences between the men and the women were soon identified, both in regard to the kinds of problems that troubled them and in their ways of coping.

At the first group meeting, while sitting in the inner circle, the fathers declared that what troubled them the most was their child's future, the shortage of qualified professional people capable of improving their child's condition, and the question: What would our lives have been like if we hadn't had this child? The mothers pointed out that the issues which most troubled them were: the child's future, a shortage of suitable educational frameworks for the child, the emotional and physical burden, fear of an additional pregnancy, their lack of social life, and their inability to go on vacation. At the beginning of the process, their mutual problems served as bridging channels, and only at the second stage was it possible to discuss the differences. A number of couples pointed out that this exercise was the first chance they had had to listen to their partner from "without" and to understand better what he or she was experiencing. Again it could be seen how defining differences can open channels for bridging them.

The discussion on intercouple relationships became temporarily an intergroup issue, so that it was removed from its specific couple-oriented context. This process contributed to the direct involvement of all the members of the group and to the sense of mutual support, which lessened the feeling of threat involved in personal revelation (Reichline and Targow, 1990). More than once, during the course of the activity, the parents asked to work in circles, especially when they felt that the differences between fathers and mothers created considerable tension between them, or when they sensed difficulties in overcoming opposing positions within the group. Slowly but surely, the gender-based circle mingled and new circles were formed based on relevant issues.

The goal of the group in terms of the exercise was, therefore, to create circles based on relevant issues and not on gender. Translated into partnership terms, the couples gained strength by separating between coping with a handicapped child and the emotional ties between them, thus creating a strong and firm emotional basis in their relationship.

Example #4: Using the DCE for Settling Conflicts:
The Case of the Interdisciplinary Team

Serious tension had arisen between the nursing and the medical teams in a specific department of a hospital. This tension upset the work routine on the ward and created an unpleasant atmosphere, causing considerable unpleasantness for the patients. The many attempts at settling the conflict between the physicians and the nurses had been unsuccessful and only made the situation worse.

One session of DCE achieved a significant breakthrough in settling the conflict. In the first stage, the doctors were asked to sit in an inner circle and to express their feelings toward their work in the department, while the nurses were listening in the outer circle. At this stage, the doctors were not permitted to refer in any way to the work of the nurses.

At the second stage, the nurses were asked to share their feelings, in the inner circle, without referring to the work of the physicians in the department, while the physicians were listening from the outer circle. The third stage consisted of a discussion, in which each speaker was asked to relate to his or her feelings "here and now."

Since the atmosphere was charged with suspicion and tension, it was very important to adhere strictly to the rules. To the surprise of the participants, it became clear during the discussion that in fact they have a great deal in common. Both physicians and nurses suffer from similar problems in their work, e.g., overwork, exhaustion, and professional decline.

In the second stage of the process the participants who felt themselves to be particularly burdened were requested to enter the inner circle. A number of physicians and nurses then entered the inner circle to discuss the reasons for this feeling of oppression and to try to uncover possible ways for alleviating it. At this stage, movement began taking place between the circles, physicians and nurses moving to and fro in accordance with their level of identification with those sitting in the inner circle. Finally a single circle was formed, united around their common problems of workload and their need to find solutions. In a discussion in the large circle, the participants reached these conclusions:

a. The reasons for the tension were not connected with being a physician or a nurse, but from pressures connected with the work environment. By recognizing this fact, it was possible to break down the professional distinctions into circles and to rebuild new circles according to relevant criteria.

b. There are more common elements between the two groups than dissimilar ones.

c. A mutual approach to solving mutual problems will turn energies in a positive direction, instead of turning them toward negative channels as in the past.

All the participants felt that the DCE had given them the opportunity to listen to the other side without the need to be defensive or to enter a struggle. Similarly, the ability to move from circle to circle allowed each of them to place themselves in a place that most expressed their feelings at the very moment. In the first stage of the exercise they felt an unbridgeable polarity. However, this polarity—expressed by the physical distancing of the physicians' circle from that of the nurses'—was responsible for making the team realize the seriousness of the situation. Once it was determined (from within this extreme conflict) that there was a great deal of common ground between them and that the reasons for the conflict were not based on belonging to one profession or the other, the way to bridging was opened, and the tension evaporated. The road was short from here to actually finding solutions to the real issues.

DISCUSSION

As the examples demonstrated, CDE makes possible an encounter between two groups of people for whom a meeting within their everyday reality would be difficult, painful, and sometimes even impossible. A safe environment is necessary for ensuring the exercise's effectiveness, although the risks involved in this exercise must also be considered.

The Strengths of DCE

First, bridging is made possible because it takes place within a training system that creates a supportive and protected environment. This support is particularly important because the introduction made between the two groups is very direct and revealing. This protection is achieved through the fact that the encounter occurs between two groups, and not between individuals and a group. This kind of encounter does not demand immediate change on the part of each participant (Blake and Mounton, 1962). Concentrating on their own behavior, and not that of their counterparts, enables members of both groups to listen and react without the need to defend themselves. A win-win situation is created.

Second, by emphasizing the differences and similarities, a swift, direct, and more revealing confrontation with the tension between the two groups is achieved. Direct confrontation permits speedy identification of possible channels for bridging: both personal and on the group level (Kernberg, 1980). By moving their seats, members of both groups are exposed to a similar process. The similar process involves an internal conflict with stereotypes and the recognition that each group is composed of individuals who are different from each other in their strengths, weaknesses, and humanness. This mutual experience stresses their similarities and opens another doorway to bridging.

Third, the system stresses the principle of equality (as opposed to philanthropy) between the two groups, thus permitting mutual mobility between them. In this way the participants are allowed free choice between the alternatives facing them and they are not obliged to conform to any predetermined mode of behavior (Rosenfeld, 1989; Blake and Mouton, 1962).

Possible Risks of the DCE

First, emphasizing the differences between the groups may create increased cohesion in each of the subgroups, producing pressure for conformity, which might prevent one or more of the participants to "cross the divide" (Heap, 1977). In other words, an individual wish for change might be construed as "betrayal" of the group, and could be left unsupported on both sides. Second, since emphasis is placed on equality between the two groups, a situation may arise where a participant in the "normal" group may cross the line to the "deviant" group. For example, a nonuser of drugs may cross over to the groups of drug addicts. Third, the confrontation between the two groups might increase the distance between them even farther. For example, to the extent of leaving the training altogether (Lewin, 1953).

All the risks mentioned here can happen in reality, as well. A qualified coordinator will encourage the groups to learn from the situation at the third step of the exercise, by helping them reflect on the common processes they were going through, thus helping to open up desired channels of bridging. This, after all, is the main objective of the exercise, with all the advantages and disadvantages inherent.

The Nature of the DCE

So far, Dynamic Circles has been referred to as an exercise, because it is guided by a coordinator during the event (Jones, 1986). What is even worse to mention is that it has several elements of simulation, too: it presents real-life situations that are translated into symbols, it has clear-cut rules and regulations, it takes place within a protected environment, and it is possible to learn relevant lessons from this technique for other real-life situations.

However, in all the examples described here, it would seem that the border between real life and simulation is often blurred. Whereas it is quite clear to pilots that they won't really crash their plane if they make mistakes during a flight simulation, it is not possible to promise the participants in a couples group that if they make a mistake, they will not have to pay a real price in couple relationship. It seems that this is the fundamental difference between simulations that demonstrate the workings of machinery and simulations that demonstrate interpersonal relationships. Simulations can reduce the price of mistakes in demonstrations of interpersonal relationships; however, they do not have the power to abolish mistakes altogether.

SUMMARY

Unlike the Fishbowl technique, the factor unique to this exercise is expressed in its physical dynamics and in its ability to conduct an ongoing group process. Its advantage lies in its ability to translate the distance between groups into visual situations, which permit group members and the coordinator to assess the changes taking place in the room at every moment and to respond to them accordingly. Forming two separate circles forces each member of each group to confront the distance between them and their feelings toward the other group, immediately and in a most direct manner. Work in the inner circle aims at clarifying these feelings in the presence of the other group without it being allowed to interfere in the larger discussion. Exposure to the other side's feelings allows members of the observing circle to feel empathy for and sometimes an affinity with the feeling being expressed by the working circle. That is to say: a positive channel for bridging has been opened, which cannot usually be opened in confrontations involving self-defense, or in a win-lose confrontation.

Finally, by comparing the way in which the groups were seated at the beginning of the exercise with the way in which they were seated at its end, both the mediator and the participants are able to evaluate the results immediately, in the most practical way.

REFERENCES

Bargal, D. and Bar, H. (1992). A Lewinian approach to intergroup workshops for Arab-Palestinian and Jewish youth. *Journal of Social Issues, 48*(2): 139-154.

Bargal, D. and Bar, H. (1994). The encounter of social selves: Intergroup workshops for Arab and Jewish youth. *Social Work with Groups, 17*(3): 39-60.

Blake, R. and Mouton, J. (1962). The intergroup dynamics of win-lose conflict and problem solving collaboration in union management relations. In J. Sherif (Ed.), *Intergroup Relations and Leadership*, New York: John-Eiley.

Chang, E.T. (1992). Building minority coalitions: A case study of Korean and African Americans, *Korea Journal of Population and Development, 21*(1): 37-56.

Crookall, D., Oxford, R., and Saunders, D. (1987). Towards a reconceptualization of simulation: From representation of reality, *Simulation/Games for Learning, 17*(4): 147-171.

Heap, K. (1977). *Group Theory for Social Workers*. New York: Pergamon Press. pp. 138-217.

Jones, K. (1986). Simulations and anxiety related to public speaking. *Simulation and Games, 17*(3): 327-344.

Johnson, D.W. and Johnson, F.P. (1991). *Joining Together: Group Theory and Group Skills*, (Fourth Edition). Englewood Cliffs, NJ, Prentice-Hall International Editors.

Kacen, L. (1998). Dynamics Circles Exercise: Intergroup bridging. *Simulation & Gaming, 29*(1): 101-104.

Kacen, L. (1998). Intergroup bridging using the Dynamic Circles Exercise (DCE). *Simulation & Gaming, 29*(1): 88-100.

Kernberg, O. (1980). *Internal World and External Reality: Object Relation Theory Applied*. New York: Jason Aronson.

Lewin, K. (1953). *A Dynamic Theory of Personality*. New York: McGraw-Hill.

Lewin, K. (1989). *Resolving Social Conflicts*. Jerusalem: Keter Publishing, (in Hebrew).

Mika, H. (Ed.) (1995). Victim and offender mediation: International perspectives on theory research and practice (special issue). *Mediation Quarterly, 12*(3).

Pfeiffer, J.W. and Jones, J.E. (1975). *Reference guide to handbooks and annuals*. CA: University Association Publishers and Consultants, p. 1.

Reichline, P.B. and Targow, J.G. (1990). Couples groups. In I.L. Kutash and A. Wolf (Eds.), *The Group Psychotherapist's Handbook, Contemporary Theory and Technique* (pp. 231-252). New York: Columbia University Press.

Rosenfeld, J.M. (1989). Emergence from extreme poverty. *Science and Service*, Paris: Fourth World Publishers, p. 17.

Rubinstein, G. (1990). Specialty vs. adaptability: Authenticity according to various therapeutic approaches. *Talks, D*(2): 95-86 (in Hebrew).

Rugel, R.P. (1991). Addictions treatment in groups: A review of therapeutic factors. *Small Group Research, 22*(4): 475-491.

Serok, S. (1980). Realizing the Gestalt theory and the establishment's approach to immigrant integration. *Society and Welfare. G*(1): 83-88 (in Hebrew).

Sherif, M. (1966). *In Common Predicament.* Boston: Houghton Mifflin.

Tajfel, H. (1982). Social psychology of intergroup relations, *Annual Review of Psychology, 33*: 1-39.

Thalhofer, N.N. (1993). Intergroup differentiation and reduction of intergroup conflict, *Small Group Research, 24*(1): 28-43.

Towle, C. (1954). The learner in education for the professions. In *Education for Social Work.* Chicago: University of Chicago Press.

Yalom, I.D. (1985). *The Theory and Practice of Group Psychotherapy* (Third Edition). New York: Basic Books Inc., p. 19.

Chapter 14

Group Work: Empowering Adults with Developmental Disabilities

Manuel Nakanishi
Phyllis Pastore

INTRODUCTION

During childhood, the participants of the program described in this chapter had been categorized by their deficits in intellectual and developmental abilities and labeled as either trainable or nontrainable, a label that can remain with them for life. This labeling process places individuals with mild and moderate developmental disabilities within the trainable classification. Unfortunately, all too often the focus of training follows *Webster's Dictionary* definition of the word trainable "to form behaviors, habits and mental attitude by discipline and instruction; to make proficient by instruction and practice." (Kellerman et al., 1981).

Therefore, the label of mild and moderate mental retardation often results in punitive treatment and subjective selection of training by care providers. The training usually focuses on behavior modification conforming with socially acceptable behavior known as social competence (Siperstein, 1992). This training results in external control because the individual receives little training geared toward achievement of cognitive understanding necessary for internalization. Furthermore, this group's early socialization occurred before laws were enacted to protect them from institutionalization or sheltered family environments that focused on their limitations. Thus, by current definition their individual and collective experiences portray oppression and disempowerment. Yet, the application of the empowerment model in working with this population is limited. Consequently, the question remains whether adults diagnosed with mild or moderate retardation can achieve internal control given the opportunity for cognitive understanding within a group setting. This question has important implications for the social work professionals who strive to ensure client-centered services for this population. It will also provide insight into the cognitive capabilities of adults in this client group.

LITERATURE

Since the mid-1960s, advocacy efforts created opportunities for children with developmental disabilities to enter services that increased their involvement in the community. Furthermore, social forces no longer sanction these children's isolation in institutional or family environments that limit their ability to achieve maximum potential. These social changes also provided opportunities for older individuals with developmental disabilities. Although once isolated and institutionalized, they now live in communities, attend sheltered workshops, and advance to community-supported employment. Nevertheless, "institutionalized or mentally retarded patients who have been isolated and enmeshed in their family have not had experiences that help them to achieve their highest potential and functioning" (Barbero, 1989, p. 546). They were socialized in roles of "passive and dependent persons, alternatively, [and] may assume the child's role that they think is expected of them" (Kaplan, Sadock, and Grebb, 1994, p. 1035). Furthermore, individuals with mental retardation are painfully aware that "they are treated differently from the way other young people are treated. Their families, their peers, and the community do not allow them to forget they are retarded." They live in a world that does to them or for them so the development of a mature value system based on internal autonomy does not occur because personal decision-making opportunities are lacking (Richards and Lee, 1972, p. 30). Gasker (1991) studied peer communication among adults with mental retardation. Her work revealed (a) expressions of solidarity and offers of help or reward are relatively infrequent among members, (b) many statements among this group are repetitive or purely observational, and (c) all verbal communication appears to occur at a far lower frequency (p. 37). Therefore, group work is important for this population. Laterza (1983) explains:

> The early socialization of the mentally retarded is often characterized by isolation inside an institution or in a sheltered home environment. The norms, values, and roles learned are limited to the attitudes expressed by significant others in their immediate surroundings. Through the small group process resocialization is taking place. These individuals are learning "selfhood" and self-realization through social connectedness. (p. 528)

This was evident in a study by Richards and Lee (1972), who used group work techniques to achieve improvement in individual self-esteem and to attain self-sustainment status in the community. Furthermore, numerous studies suggest the usefulness of groups for skill acquisition by this population. Lee and Lee (1989) found that students between the ages of fourteen and twenty-one are highly capable of learning age-appropriate behaviors, becoming more expressive, contributing their own ideas to the group process, and feeling better about themselves. Blistein (1992) reported social group treatment successfully assisted dually diagnosed adults to change narcissistic behavior and thus achieve team spirit in a group home setting. Lee (1977) used a group program to enhance social adjustment skills of institutionalized adults with moderate mental retardation. His program consisted of thirty sessions designed to improve social interaction, personal appearance and mannerisms, awareness of feelings, making friends, and social responsibility. The result of his program showed a significant change in four of the five areas and a surprisingly significant improvement in associative verbal intelligence.

Another group study conducted by Fine, Tangeman, and Woodard (1990) assessed the changes in adaptive behavior of older adults with mental retardation following deinstitutionalization. They found increased adaptive behavior and improvements in economic activity, language development, and domestic activity. In addition, their study found an increase in adaptive behavior that could be explained by the increased opportunity for interaction with staff and other adults. Bates (1980) also studied interpersonal skills training for acquiring social skills by this population. His study found that adults with mental retardation could gain new skills after twelve training sessions. Sherman and colleagues (1992) conducted a study to evaluate social skills by comparing performances of people with and without mental retardation. Their results found adults with mental retardation scored similarly to members of the community in following instructions and accepting criticism, but lower on negotiation skills.

As the above studies indicate, individuals with developmental disabilities continue to learn new skills if given the opportunity; however, their chances for achieving empowerment and internalizing control continue to be limited. This is explained by Black and Weiss (1991) as the "social construction of disability":

> . . . people with chronic illness and disabilities share the sociological situation of discrimination in our society and therefore should be viewed as an oppressed minority group. This oppression takes such forms as outright prejudice, job discrimination and misconceptions that exaggerate the true limitations of a given handicap (Gliedman and Roth, 1980). [Also], . . . to the extent that disabled persons and their families share society's discriminatory views of handicapped persons, they are likely to experience greater personal difficulty and to feel less hopeful about the future. (pp. 138-139)

Therefore, this oppressed population needs empowerment and peer group interaction to acquire the decision-making skills necessary for internalizing control. Also, an empowerment approach to the group may have further positive results for this population by enabling them to request needed and desired services.

THE SETTING

The agency is a private, not-for-profit organization serving adults with physical, mental, emotional, and medical disabilities. Its primary focus is vocational training. At the time of the study, the agency had 157 clients of which 127 were diagnosed with mild, moderate, or severe mental retardation. The remaining thirty clients were diagnosed within several classification categories including cerebral palsy, spina bifida, Down's syndrome, epilepsy, brain damage, depression, schizoaffective disorder, and schizophrenia. However, most of the clients had multiple diagnoses and could be placed in several classification categories. The client's contractual agreement offers individual and group counseling by a staff social worker or any student intern currently at the agency.

AIM

The study was designed to investigate the effectiveness of a supportive empowering milieu for increasing individual group members' (a) self-expression, (b) self-esteem, and (c) self-control, by providing opportunistic social interactions to heighten cognitive awareness and growth for adults with developmental disabilities. Therefore, based on the group member's past socialization, the worker's intervention required both actual decision-making opportunities and tasks to increase cognitive understanding of self-control. This is explained by Siperstein (1992) as social competence [that] reflects the marriage of social knowledge (social cognition) and social action (social behavior) (p. iv). The social worker defined increased self-expression as both personal verbalization and personal interaction within the group. Also, an increase of self-control was defined in terms of self-generated reductions in inappropriate behaviors and lengthened task performance resulting in increased wages.

THEORETICAL FRAMEWORK

An empowerment approach described by Dunst, Trivette, and Deal (1988) and Rappaport (1985) was applied. This approach defines the group leader's role as both proactive and enabling because the empowering relationship is built on the following: (a) the client is already competent or has the capacity to become competent in the skill, (b) failure to display competency originates in the social system by failing to provide opportunities for expression, and (c) the client develops an understanding that he or she can change behavior to gain control (p. 4). This approach focuses on the strengths of clients rather than their deficits, and it represents an alternative perspective not normally applied to this special population. Furthermore, the group worker incorporated several empowerment concepts outlined by Lee (1994; 1983), Lee and Lee (1989), and Cowger (1994). First, the worker focused on developing a partnership with the group and fostered equal dialogue between the worker and members. Second, the worker understood that ownership of the group belonged to the group members. Furthermore, the worker used questions to enter the member's world, stimulate dialogue, and promote group cohesion.

THE GROUP

The open-ended group consisted of fifteen to eighteen clients of both genders, diagnosed with mild or moderate mental retardation; however, many of these clients had multiple diagnostic classifications. The members ranged in age from twenty-four to sixty-four and lived in either group homes or with their parent(s). Their length of time at the agency ranged from one to six years.

Upon entering the group, the worker's initial assessment found little interaction among the members, with most of the interaction consisting of derogatory name-calling. All authority remained with the leader. The group itself had no direction or purpose, and the members were not sure why they were attending the group except that they were told to come. Therefore, the group process was not helping the clients learn resocialization as described by Laterza (1983). Furthermore, lack of concern for the group's development and the fact that group members lost pay as a result of attending group sessions demonstrated limitation and disempowerment of clients within the agency.

THE PROCESS

The program application was divided into two four-week stages based on the socialization and communication patterns of this special population. The main goal of the first stage was to resocialize the members to value self-expression and group interaction by achieving cohesiveness. The worker used questions and actively demonstrated verbal and nonverbal listening skills to seek a response from each group member. These techniques were selected based on the worker's beliefs and understanding of the empowerment process. First, it validated the members' worth, both personally and in the group itself. Second, both the verbal and nonverbal message sent by the worker portrayed the idea that self-expression is both appropriate and valued.

Initially questions such as "Tell me something about you" or "Why are you in the group?" were used for their general nature; nevertheless, these questions provided valuable insight into the members' world. Furthermore, their geniality allowed the decision-making process to start in a comfortable manner. The worker continued using questions until all group members freely volunteered a response. However, two critical issues in the use of questions must be addressed and explained. First, the worker demonstrated acceptance and validated the member's decision regardless of whether the member decided to respond or not. This empowered the members to make decisions and increased their skill in this ability. Second, the worker recognized and accepted the different communication patterns used by members within the group and the worker aligned her communication style to fit the group. The group members' communication patterns individually and collectively required more time for analyzing and responding to information and questions. Their response time might be a minute or two longer than the worker's, so the worker empowered them by demonstrating patience.

If the group worker fails to understand this point, the group members can become confused, frustrated, and withdrawn. Therefore, group workers need to continually monitor their actions and avoid seeking a response within their own communication pattern when working with this special population. This process actually results in a resocialization for both the members and the worker.

Also, based on the worker's initial assessment of the group, the first four sessions were ended with a request that all members join hands and repeat: "We wish each other a happy and healthy week."

This was used to aid group development, cohesiveness, and social interactions.

The main goal of the second stage was to provide the opportunity for self-generated expression and request. Therefore, the worker needed to eliminate asking the group questions; however, the empowerment process required two additional questions to be addressed. Thus, at the start of the fifth session the worker asked the group members these questions: "What do you not like about being here?" and "What changes would you make?" These questions created the turning point for the group because the members had never before been given the opportunity to address these issues. At first the questions were answered with requests for sports equipment and more time off from their jobs for fun. However, several group members addressed the issue of their worth at the agency. In addition, when the worker ended this session the group members self-directed the closing as outlined previously.

During the remaining sessions of this stage, the worker not only became part of the group, but the members achieved self-direction. The group selected a name for themselves based on members' suggestions. They agreed on the name "Support Group," and identified their purpose as "helping new people in the agency so they don't feel alone." The members asked questions, sought help, and expressed feeling within the group setting. They expressed concern when a member missed a session, and they established their own norms within the group.

EXTENDED ACTIVITIES

Several weeks into this program, changes started to occur outside the group setting as well. First, the group worker was informed that several group members and nongroup members requested a self-directed holiday party. The agency staff was surprised by their request but eventually agreed to it. The party was described by both clients and staff as the best one in the history of the agency. Next, the group worker was summoned to the lunchroom by one of the client's vocational instructors. Upon arriving in the room the instructor pointed to three group members and stated, "Look at what they did." At the instruction of the agency director, the lunchroom tables are separated to allow a maximum of four individuals to sit together; however, that day three group members had rearranged several tables in the room to form one large group of sixteen. The instructor reported that in his five years at the agency he never witnessed this action by clients. The members continued to rearrange the tables from that day forward. This action reflects an extension and individualization of the empowerment process occurring with the group.

SUMMARY AND IMPLICATIONS

Each member of the group increased both their verbalization and interaction within the group. They gained a sense of power in understanding their self-control. Their cognitive awareness was demonstrated by increased task performance and wages.

Implications

As a result of this study the worker realized that for this special population "(s)ociety's responses to the people in this population have a fundamental impact on their daily lives and on the development of their potential" (Black and Weiss, 1991, p. 162). Furthermore, as explained by Brantley and Gemmill (1990) "Persons with mental retardation require a diversity of services, and social workers' major role is the provision and coordination of the service" (p. 284)." This includes services offered within an agency as well. Also, the worker realized the tremendous personal and professional growth that occurred by both the process itself and the opportunity to work with this special group.

Recommendations

It is strongly recommended that this special population be given the opportunity to achieve their highest level of potential. Furthermore, the social work profession must guard against underestimating this population due to their complacency with authority figures based on their early socialization. Finally, it is recommended that this process be utilized to empower this special population so that they can indeed become active participants in society.

REFERENCES

Barbero, S.L. (1989). Community-based, day treatment for mentally retarded adults. *Social Work, 34*(6): 545-548.

Bates, P. (1980). The effectiveness of interpersonal skills training on the social skill acquisition of moderately and mildly retarded adults. *Journal of Applied Behavior Analysis, 13*(2): 237-248.

Black, R.B. and Weiss, J.O. (1991). Chronic physical illness and disability. In A. Gitterman (Ed.), *Handbook of Social Work Practice with Vulnerable Populations* (pp. 137-164). New York: Columbia University Press.

Blistein, S. (1992). Life with the H-team: From narcissism to team spirit: Social group treatment for the dually diagnosed in group homes. *Social Work with Groups, 15*(2/3): 37-51.

Brantley, D.M. and Gemmill, P.A. (1990). Mental retardation. In A. Gitterman (Ed.), *Handbook of Social Work Practice with Vulnerable Populations* (265-285). New York: Columbia University Press.

Cowger, C.D. (1994). Assessing client strengths: Clinical assessment for client empowerment. *Social Work, 39*(3): 262-268.

Dunst, C., Trivette, D., and Deal, A. (1988). *Enabling and Empowering Families: Principles and Guidelines for Practice.* Cambridge, MA: Brookline Books.

Fine, M.A., Tangeman, P.J., and Woodard, J. (1990). Changes in adaptive behaviors of older adults with mental retardation following deinstitutionalization. *American Journal on Mental Retardation, 94*(6): 661-668.

Gasker, J.A. (1991). Peer communication among adults with mental retardation in a community setting: Patterns and intervention strategies. *Adult Residential Care Journal, 5*(1): 29-43.

Kaplan, H.I., Sadock, B.J., and Grebb, J.A. (1994). *Kaplan and Sadock's Synopsis of Psychiatry: Behavioral Sciences, Clinical Psychiatry* (Seventh Edition) Baltimore, MD: Williams and Wilkins.

Kellerman, D.F. et al. (Eds.) (1981). *The Webster Reference Dictionary of the English Language* (Encyclopedic Edition, Volumes 1-2). Baltimore, MD: United Guild.

Laterza, P. (1983). An eclectic approach to group work with mentally retarded. In F.J. Turner (Ed.), *Differential Diagnosis and Treatment in Social Work* (pp. 520-529). New York: Free Press.

Lee, D.Y. (1977). Evaluation of a group-counseling program designed to enhance social adjustment of mentally retarded adults. *Journal of Counseling Psychology, 24*(4): 318-323.

Lee, J.A. (1983). The group: A chance at human connection for the mentally impaired older person. *Social Work with Groups, 5*(2): 43-55.

Lee, J.A.B. (1994). *The empowerment approach to social work practice.* New York: Columbia University Press.

Lee, B. and Lee, S. (1989). Group therapy as a process to strengthen the independence of students with mental retardation. *Social Work in Education, 11*(2): 123-132.

Rappaport, J. (1985). The power of empowerment language. *Social Policy*, Fall, 15-21.

Richards, L.D. and Lee, K.A. (1972). Group process in social habilitation of the retarded. *Social Casework, 53*(1): 30-37.

Sherman, J.A., Sheldon, J.B., Harchik, A.E., Edwards, K., and Quinn, J.M. (1992). Social evaluation of behaviors comprising three social skills and a comparison of the performance of people with and without mental retardation. *American Journal on Mental Retardation, 96*(4): 419-432.

Siperstein, G.N. (1992). Social competence: An important construct in mental retardation. *American Journal on Mental Retardation, 96*(4): iii-vi.

Index

Order Your Own Copy of
This Important Book for Your Personal Library!

REBUILDING COMMUNITIES
Challenges for Group Work

_____in hardbound at $39.95 (ISBN: 0-7890-0722-3)

_____in softbound at $24.95 (ISBN: 0-7890-0942-0)

COST OF BOOKS_____

OUTSIDE USA/CANADA/
MEXICO: ADD 20%_____

POSTAGE & HANDLING_____
*(US: $3.00 for first book & $1.25
for each additional book)
Outside US: $4.75 for first book
& $1.75 for each additional book)*

SUBTOTAL_____

IN CANADA: ADD 7% GST_____

STATE TAX_____
*(NY, OH & MN residents, please
add appropriate local sales tax)*

FINAL TOTAL_____
*(If paying in Canadian funds,
convert using the current
exchange rate. UNESCO
coupons welcome.)*

☐ **BILL ME LATER:** ($5 service charge will be added)
(Bill-me option is good on US/Canada/Mexico orders only;
not good to jobbers, wholesalers, or subscription agencies.)

☐ Check here if billing address is different from
shipping address and attach purchase order and
billing address information.

Signature _____

☐ **PAYMENT ENCLOSED: $**_____

☐ **PLEASE CHARGE TO MY CREDIT CARD.**

☐ Visa ☐ MasterCard ☐ AmEx ☐ Discover
☐ Diner's Club

Account # _____

Exp. Date _____

Signature _____

Prices in US dollars and subject to change without notice.

NAME _____

INSTITUTION _____

ADDRESS _____

CITY _____

STATE/ZIP _____

COUNTRY _____ COUNTY (NY residents only) _____

TEL _____ FAX _____

E-MAIL_____
May we use your e-mail address for confirmations and other types of information? ☐ Yes ☐ No

Order From Your Local Bookstore or Directly From
The Haworth Press, Inc.
10 Alice Street, Binghamton, New York 13904-1580 • USA
TELEPHONE: 1-800-HAWORTH (1-800-429-6784) / Outside US/Canada: (607) 722-5857
FAX: 1-800-895-0582 / Outside US/Canada: (607) 772-6362
E-mail: getinfo@haworthpressinc.com
PLEASE PHOTOCOPY THIS FORM FOR YOUR PERSONAL USE.

BOF96

DATE DUE
